ADRIENNE J. GOODMAN-LAMORA, DACM, L.AC.

Balance Is A Wild Goose Chase

Why Women Should Focus More On Nourishment and Moderation To Achieve Wellness

First published by Wild Goose Press 2021

Acknowledgements to the proof readers: Judy Fletcher, Wendy Chudner, Deborah Vanderpool, Brooke Castrechini, Kim Day, Christine Poole, Sherrie DiStefano. (Thank you!!!)

First edition

ISBN: 978-1-7368129-0-7

This book was professionally typeset on Reedsy.
Find out more at reedsy.com

Contents

II   The Physical Needs of Women

III   Women's Mental & Emotional Health

Dedication

To all of my patients over the years.
You've taught me more than I could have ever imagined possible.

To my husband Matt.
You always believe in me, encourage me and give me the space I need to open my wings.
For that, I am forever grateful.

THANK YOU.

I

Introduction

Are You Nourished?

As women, we all desire to be "healthy," don't we? To spend our days feeling energetic, productive, content, worry and pain-free? The barriers lie *not* in trying (we are all trying our best), but in not *knowing* what to do or how to fit it in, and in battling our tendencies towards self-sabotage. We can't truly be "well" (or nourished, as I call it) unless we are taking care of our WHOLE self.. not just the physical parts, but the mental and emotional parts, too.

After many years of treating women (and knowing them!), I see that **most** women struggle with chronic, poorly managed physical, mental and emotional issues, and I know why. It's because we were never taught how to properly care for ourselves, and we've been fed misinformation: information based on male physiology, NOT female physiology. We are expected to function like men, and men we are not! We have been taught to use unhealthy coping mechanisms in an attempt to conform to what we think we "should" be or do. If we, as women, want to be (and continue to be) strong, healthy and nourished, then this has to STOP. The sooner the better!

How often do we ask ourselves "Is my body properly nourished"? That's kind of a LOL question, right? Uh, like never? So we grow up going to the doctor for "check ups" and we undergo a series of tests to make sure that all of our systems are running as expected. Your weight is assessed, your urine is tested, the doctor runs a series of tests by looking, listening, and feeling. You'll likely send you out to have blood drawn so more tests can be run. Most patients have no idea what any of the tests are for. This is the gold standard for the general Western medical exam, which most Americans have come to rely upon as their gauge of "health and wellbeing." I'm here to tell you that this is NOT a good gauge. If you are reading this, you probably already know that. Yes, at the basic level, it means that all the systems that keep you alive are functioning. So, you get to continue to be "alive" in the physical sense of the word. The issue is that there is a HUGE gap between physically being *alive* and living a happy and healthy life. I'm here to help you bridge the gap between the two. My particular focus is on women because in my experience as a Doctor of Chinese medicine, women struggle with the latter. A LOT. Physically AND mentally.

As a general statement from my personal and professional experience, most women in the U.S. are undernourished and as a result, are struggling with poorly managed physical, mental and emotional health conditions. I think it's very hard to be a woman in today's Western society. We are constantly judged, no matter what choices we make and we never feel like what we do is good enough. There isn't enough time in a day to pursue both what we want, and to keep up with all the things we think we "should" be doing from a cultural standpoint. We are even judged by our own smart watches! Therefore, we are the population that is most susceptible to depression, anxiety, stress, sleep issues, heart disease, menstrual issues, etc, and all the while, we continue to care for our families, friends, households, careers, ourselves and often are the ones who maintain order in our chaotic lives. The very reason that we end up suffering from one or more of the conditions I listed above is that we are overworked and stressed, and we do not nourish ourselves properly. Either we do not know how, or we do not *allow* ourselves the time to take care for ourselves properly. In turn, we cannot offset the rigor of our daily, weekly, yearly lives. Is it any wonder that by the time we reach menopause, we are irritable, exhausted, in chronic pain, can't sleep and suffer from all kinds of uncomfortable ailments? Let me ask you this question: What happens to your car when you run it and continue to run it without putting oil in it? Everyone knows what happens then! Just like with your vehicle, your body will begin to break down if you are running it hard and not putting in what it needs to function properly. It may still pass that general inspection when the time comes, but that doesn't mean it is actually working as well as it could. One of the biggest problems in our medical culture is that we are not taught the importance of maintaining our bodies as clearly as we are taught to maintain our vehicles! Crazy, right?!

Giving our bodies what they *physically* need isn't the only issue, is it? We are bombarded with information on how to eat healthy and exercise: what we "should" or "should not" eat, "should" or "should not" do. If every woman could just start eating healthy and exercise, problem solved, right? Ah! If only it were that simple. The problem is that we are still struggling with finding balance, even more so when you add the stress of healthy eating and exercise into lives that are already bursting at the seams. The thing is, we are much more complex than a car. We are extremely complex beings. Far more complex than a 5 minute exam at the doctor's office is going to be able to assess. That isn't even enough to assess our purely physical wellbeing. We have a whole mental and emotional side of us that go largely untreated! We have ruminating thoughts, guilt and have habits that we use to soothe our stress that are counterproductive to our goals. We sabotage our own efforts to make changes because we have never learned to actually care for our entire being, to assure that both our physical and mental selves are nourished. In not doing that, we have created unhealthy coping mechanisms that many of us have to either learn how to avoid or undo altogether. Undoing is harder and will take more time, if it is even entirely possible.

It's OK!! All of this is completely normal. Most of us women are in the exact same boat. I'm here to tell you that you can still lead a more fulfilling and healthy life while not being perfectly happy and healthy ALL THE TIME. Why do I know that? I know that because I am one of you. I'm a mom, a wife, a doctor of Chinese Medicine, a teacher, an author and an athlete. I struggle every day with taking care of myself: physically, mentally and emotionally, all while battling my own unproductive habits and tendencies. I am going to offer you information about what your physical, mental and emotional body needs to function more efficiently, along with tips on how to accomplish it. It may seem overwhelming, depending on how much of this knowledge you already possess. The aim of this book is to give you all the tools necessary to work towards not only physical wellness, but also mental and emotional

5

wellness. The physical body can't be "healthy" if our minds are tormented and unsettled by disruptive thoughts, and if we are continuously using unhealthy coping mechanisms to deal with life. In Chinese medicine, the body and mind are **not** separate entities. This is a purely Western idea, and its creation and existence have been extremely detrimental to the health and wellbeing of those of us living in the West. Ironically, it has actually put us *behind* the curve in terms of health.

The reason I wrote this book is because the advice I have to offer women about improving their health, and ultimately, their lives, is extensive. It's far more complicated than what I can cover in an appointment, a few appointments, or even a short article or video. There can never be enough time to help as much as I want to. I knew I needed to write an entire *book* about it. The key to prolonged wellness is about **everything** you do. What you eat, how/if you move, your sleep, your thoughts and internal dialogue, your decisions, your activities, your relationships, your attitude towards yourself and others! An improvement in any of these areas is going to help overall. So I decided to cover what I think are the most important points, and still I know I have missed some. All I can hope for is that even the tiniest piece of this book helps at least some women in some way.. we could all use it.. and we all deserve to take better care of ourselves!

Moderation is Key

My favorite thing about Chinese medicine (which is based on traditional Chinese culture) is that nothing in life is "black and white," and everything around us and inside of us is interconnected. For example, our bodies and minds are not separate entities. They are intertwined and the state of one affects the state of the other. One of the biggest topics in Chinese medicine is the ancient concept of "moderation". This is a really profound concept that seems to have been lost on us Americans as we are always striving for more, more, more! Mirriam-Webster dictionary defines the word *moderation* as "in a way that is reasonable and not excessive." Moderation is considered a key part of one's personal development in Chinese Taoist philosophy and religion.

> *"Everything in moderation,*
> *even moderation."*
> *- Oscar Wilde*

One of the fundamental ideas behind Chinese medicine, which is the basis of what I teach my patients and how I try to live my own life, is that most things are OK in moderation. Even healthy behaviors can be damaging when they are done in excess: for example, even excessive food restriction and excessive exercise can damage the body over time. On the flip side, most behaviors that are considered "unhealthy" are really not overly damaging unless they are done in excess, and repeatedly over time. Our bodies are amazing! They can adapt, heal and recover like nothing I've ever seen.. but you have to give them the time and resources to do so. The problems arise when the abusive behaviors occur in excess, and are not balanced out by behaviors that support healing and recovery of the body.

Consider the paradox of lung cancer rates in Japan. It has been well known for a long time, that even though cigarette smoking is just as common in Japan and other Asian countries as it is in the United States, their risk for developing lung cancer is far lower than it is in this country. While the reason for this has not been fully proven, it is surmised that the lower incidence is related to the differences in lifestyle, diet or possibly environmental factors. Clearly, whatever they are doing, they are engaging in behaviors outside of smoking that are allowing their bodies to offset the negative effects of smoking, so the smoking is not taking a cumulative effect on the body. What those behaviors actually are, are still in question. They could be cultural, environmental, diet and lifestyle behaviors, a combination.

So, what's my point here? My point is that our bodies are resilient and while I am not suggesting that you should engage in unhealthy behaviors if you can help it, I feel that it is better to not let them be a total roadblock to making changes in other areas of your life. If you think that a smoker can't run a 5k, think again. Did you know there's a whole community of runners that think it's fun to smoke marijuana and then go out for a run? I read an article on *Runner's World* about it. And speaking of runners, having been in the athlete community for quite some time, I can assure you that athletic social activities often involve alcohol as a reward after a run or race, and even sometimes during the race. Meeting for early morning workouts with a hangover is a common occurrence!

If you think your diet is derailing your progress but you don't want to part with certain foods, there are solutions to that too. If you are having trouble eating healthy because you get constant sugar cravings, then promise yourself a healthy meal before the sugary snack or try to eat the sugary snack in *moderation*. If you can't, there may be other factors at play. Moderation often requires discipline and consistency, but it's totally doable. And it offers you a reward system for doing something that maybe you're not quite feeling like doing at the moment.

Moderation in some areas of my life does NOT come naturally for me.. obviously.. why else would I choose to do such a crazy thing as a full distance triathlon? I can certainly be an extremist in some areas of my life, and so I consciously have to mentally work to keep some things in check. Moderation can be difficult to maintain from time to time, but what is important is that you check yourself now and again, acknowledge that you've slid too far off to one side and make an effort to bring things back into balance.. at least for a little while. More than likely, things will eventually slide out again and you will have to repeat the process over and over again.. but that is normal! Moderation doesn't mean that everything is balanced ALL THE TIME. It's an AVERAGE. It's an "ebb and flow," and it WILL change with the seasons, with life changes, with hormonal changes. We have to learn to "ride the wave."

We all have our vices and our reasons for purposely engaging in behaviors that we know are not in the best interests of our health. Some of the reasons are so ingrained in us that we can't even consciously figure out why we are doing it despite the attempt to do so. In my opinion, it is STILL better to work around and with them, then to just give up and not bother trying at all. Engaging in healthy behaviors can help to offset some of the damage being created by the "bad" habits.

Our Vices/"Unhealthy" Habits

I come from families on both sides where alcohol use and abuse were common. Both my parents struggled with overusing alcohol at certain times in their lives. In addition, both my parents were smokers while I was growing up. My mom even continued to smoke while I was in utero, which is taboo now but was fairly common at the time. It's probably safe to say that I exited the womb with a predilection towards alcohol and tobacco. I started smoking cigarettes around age 13 and starting drinking alcohol shortly after that. I spent my teens, twenties and even thirties and early forties drinking socially and too often, drinking too much. Somewhere around my mid-20s, after I had graduated with my Bachelors Degree and gained about 30 pounds in the process, I became obsessed with working out and eating healthy and even dabbled a bit in competitive bodybuilding. I did have to give up drinking while dieting for the bodybuilding shows, but I never gave up smoking. I remember sneaking out the back door at one of the bodybuilding shows and smoking a cigarette. Here I was, in the best shape of my life, smoking a cigarette outside the back door of a bodybuilding competition! I felt like a total hypocrite. I did finally stop smoking when I found out I was pregnant with my daughter, and I didn't smoke again for 3 years, after I left my daughter's father and started going out socially on the nights when I was alone. This is also, not surprisingly, when my drinking also ramped up again. It took me until I entered my 40s to finally come to terms with the fact that I have some social anxiety, and I often use drinking as a means to dampen that anxiety. Occasionally, I would go overboard and end up too drunk at a family or social gathering. I also really like to smoke cigarettes when I drink so more drinking means more smoking. I did remarry, and my husband is very sociable, so I find myself in social situations much more often, and this is something I have had to grapple with. Basically, in a nutshell, I work hard regularly to keep the drinking and smoking under control and it isn't always an easy task. Sometimes it takes over, ebbs and flows, but I have also started to realize that I'm not a bad person, and I'm not a hypocrite, I'm just doing my best to deal with strong forces that sometimes take on a life of their own. I'm 42 now. You'd think it would get easier, but sometimes it seems to only get harder. Habits can be VERY difficult to change! It seems like I spent the first 20 years of my life developing bad ones and the last 20 years trying to undo them!

So now that I have spilled all of that, I can also tell you that I consider myself to be quite accomplished. I have a Bachelors Degree in Computer Engineering. I entered the workforce at age 24 as a software engineer, making great money for someone my age, but I was totally unfulfilled. The birth of my daughter at age 30 sent me into a tailspin as I couldn't stand to be away from her, much less while doing a job that I felt sucked the life out of me. I chucked all my engineering plans out the window, and went back to school for Acupuncture & Oriental Medicine, health was where my passion was anyways, much to the dismay of my ex-husband. That decision pretty much broke the already tenuous marriage, and I decided to head for the hills when my daughter was 3 and I was still a full-time student. I received my Masters Degree in 2011, opened my own acupuncture practice, which I successfully built from scratch into a thriving practice. In 2015, I married the love of my life. I started teaching at the local acupuncture college in 2017. In 2019, I completed my Doctorate, decided to train for a full distance triathlon and wrote this book. I am a proud mom of an amazing and well-adjusted 12 year old, and I do my best to be there and to support her in her many activities, and I think I do a good job at that! I eat well and I am in great shape, and sometimes I drink too much and sometimes I smoke too much. But you know what? I actually got the idea for this book while doing the last two by a campfire with my husband. (The topic was his idea.)

So the real reason I told you all that is this: this is stuff no one really talks about, and I think it is because people are ashamed of it, especially people who live an otherwise healthy life. I find that men are more willing to admit to having unhealthy habits than women. As women, we often place the ideal of being "perfect" on ourselves, and then beat ourselves up when we are not. I know that I have done the same many, many, many times. Unfortunately, beating ourselves up is counterproductive and often leads to us engaging in more of the unhealthy behavior to soothe the fact that we feel like crap about ourselves. What really needs to happen is that we need to accept it for what it is and move on. This isn't to say that working to cut back or to quit whatever you are doing isn't in your best interest, because it probably is, but I know just as well as anyone that it can be far more complicated than that.

So what are the things that you do that annoy you most, that you feel like you really "should" give up, but just don't for whatever reason? Too much time on social media? You worry too much about what other people think, to the point that it stops you from doing what you really want to be doing? Chemical addictions, like alcohol, nicotine, marijuana or other drugs? Overeating? Procrastinating?

Clearly, some of these subjects are more taboo than others, and people certainly seem to be more ashamed of chemical addictions than of being addicted to social media. I was curious to see how many would publicly come clean about these behaviors, so I posted a poll on my Facebook page, of which I have about 560 some odd Facebook "friends". I asked people to kindly share what behaviors they engage in that they know are "unhealthy" or find interfere with their ability to accomplish the things they want to get done. I received around 20 responses, mostly revolving around too much social media, TV, procrastination and eating. That leaves a lot of people who aren't comfortable publicly admitting to any more serious offenses than that. I was disappointed to see that such a small number of people responded, and admitted only to the more "cultural acceptable" offenses. This leads me to believe that people are ashamed to publicly admit other behaviors for fear of judgement, and I find that heartbreaking.

I know from my own personal experiences that alcohol abuse is rampant, yet people are hard pressed to admit they drink too much. Culturally, it's an easy thing to abuse and it is even socially acceptable. On the other hand, smoker shaming has become trendy, which has forced a lot of people to become "closet smokers" or vapers (which we have found out is way more harmful). Wasting tons of time and ignoring responsibilities, friends and family while scrolling through social media is now the "in" thing to do, and using marijuana is starting to get there too.

In any case, *everyone* struggles with keeping bad habits under control, even those of us who seem to have it all together. Beating yourself up over these things actually makes things WORSE for you, and not better. Only when you accept it, accept who you are and what you need, will you be able to move on. Sometimes I don't actually have it all together.. I am human, and I succumb to them too, but fighting these habits and feeling bad about yourself only gives them more power over you. So for now, let's just let that stuff go. Be forgiving and stop beating yourself up! We are complex beings and we do things that go even beyond the realm of our own understanding of ourselves.. crazy, but true!! Let's first start figuring out ways to make improvements in other areas of our lives, areas that we feel are easier for us to make changes. If thinking about changing or giving up something specific makes you feel stressed, start with something else. Let's focus on the positive and NOT the negative.

Letting Go Of Expectations

"Expectation is the root of all heartache."
-Shakespeare

Expectations are our biggest barrier to getting to where we want to be. Just like bad habits, we all have expectations. About everything. Even when we don't realize that we do. Expectations are unconsciously placed in our minds by everyone around us. They date back to the day we were born. Our family unit usually becomes the "normal", and if it doesn't, it may be something else that we see or hear other people doing that does. The fact that the word "normal" exists at all is evidence of our expectations. What exactly is "normal", and what, for crying out loud, is the definition of the word "good"?! What constitutes a "good" person? A "good" boy? A "good" girl? A "good" restaurant? A "good" doctor? Isn't that term completely subjective and matter of opinion? Yet, have you ever noticed how *frequently* that word is used when describing people? Isn't it an ideal that we all aspire to, even though we cannot even define it? I despise that word when it comes to describing people. It represents the epitome of expectation.

I've had my own expectations that I've needed work through. I *expected* that when I got a degree, got a job, got married, bought a house, and had a baby that I would be happy. I wasn't. Isn't that what everyone does? I *expected* that I would naturally lose some weight that I had gained while training 2-4 hours a day for my Ironman. Seems logical right? Didn't happen.

Let me preface this by saying that this isn't to account for situations where things happen outside of our control, but for the situations where we create suffering in our own minds for the simple fact that we *expected* things to be or to turn out differently. We mourn divorces and feel like failures when we find out that things didn't turn out as we *expected*. We get angry and frustrated with people because they didn't act the way we *expected* they should or would. We don't even bother signing up for that Couch To 5K program because we *expect* that people who are overweight can't run 3 miles, or we *expect* that people are going to laugh if we fail. Chances are, it's your expectations that are actually holding you back, not others or your habits. Successful people come in all colors, shapes and sizes, from the inside out.

Have you ever taken a few minutes to think about whether expectations you have are holding you back? If you haven't, I would definitely suggest that you take some time to do so. It can be a game changer!

If you have never read *"The Four Agreements: A Practical Guide to Personal Freedom (A Toltec Wisdom Book)"*, by Don Miguel Ruiz.. I absolutely recommend that you do. You'll thank me! It is small, but mighty!

Getting Out of Your Comfort Zone

"Your life does not get better by chance,
it gets better by change."
– Jim Rohn

O ne of our most limiting behaviors as human beings is our resistance and utter fear of being uncomfortable, whether it be physically or emotionally, and this fear often keeps us locked into our usual activities and routines. When we are only engaging in activities and making decisions based on our comfort level, we are not making any changes. We are not inviting anything new into our lives, and so it is not a wonder when nothing changes. In order to change, you have to create a shift within your life and it is quite possible that this shift is going to be a little uncomfortable for awhile until you acclimate to it. Luckily, this process is only temporary and you will find your new level of "normal" in no time. As human beings, we are excellent at adapting.

The hardest part of change is actually just initiating it. Getting your mindset right, and then just *doing* it. Even rules in physics state that the greatest force is needed to get an object moving in the first place, and that less force is needed to KEEP the object moving. The same concept applies to eliciting change in your life. People put off making changes for days, months, and even years but find that once they make that final decision and get started, that keeping it going is far easier. But we procrastinate simply out of fear of being uncomfortable.

The most interesting part of all this is that our fear initially contains us to a small circle or a "bubble," as I like to call it. The fear that we feel is a defense mechanism created by our subconscious for the purpose of self-preservation. Instinctually, our minds respond to changes in our comfort level and they throw up red flags when we get uneasy. I suppose that many experts attribute this to our innate "animal" instincts, that "fight or flight" response that used to rule our prehistoric ancestors, and that noticeable response you see in animals when they get spooked. However, we are a much more complex and evolved species, and most of us don't have to worry about defending our lives on a daily basis. Yet the fear response is still strong, and in many people, it actually guides their decisions.

Fear and expectations govern the perimeter of that "bubble," aka: your comfort zone. The size of the bubble depends on a number of factors: social, cultural and biological. Some people seem to be inherently more fearful than others, and some have fear and limitations placed on them as a result of their upbringing, solidified by their social and cultural surroundings. What we don't inherently realize is that this line that confines us doesn't even really exist, except in our own minds. It is entirely possible to cross it in most cases - it WILL be uncomfortable - but the thing is, when you actually step outside that bubble, you'll find a whole new world out there! You'll be amazed at how big your world gets when you continue to step outside and break through the barriers that were seemingly holding you in there. You will find people in your new world too, people who would have never met otherwise, people who have had the courage to knock down their own walls, people who share your struggles and who maybe have similar interests, goals and dreams.

Some people are seemingly OK with staying within the confines of their bubble. Others, like me, are constantly stomping down the perimeter to see just how flimsy or rigid it really is, and I have certainly fought my way through both kinds. The emotional barriers are the hardest ones for me to get through, and there are still some that I haven't managed to knock down, but I am always working towards self-awareness and self-improvement.

It's probably safe to say that I've actually become a little bit of a "change" junkie, as I have become addicted to the excitement that comes with doing things that I have never done before. I now purposely agree to do things that intimidate me or make me uncomfortable. Monotony makes me insane. Yes, it's scary and even downright terrifying at times, but the sheer elation that comes from accomplishing something that was seemingly out of my reach before makes the whole "uncomfortable" part seem worth it in the end. But that's just it. You have to persevere and get to the end (or at least far enough down the road to be able to look back) in order to see that it was all worth it. Sometimes you just have to set off down the road and have faith, and that is downright terrifying for most people.

If you haven't made sense out of anything I've said, then I will give you an example from my own life, and maybe that will set you straight. I have many examples, but for some reason I really like the story about my long and windy path to becoming a "swimmer." Of the many journeys I have made in my life, becoming adept and comfortable swimming in open water is one that I am most proud of. I think it's because it's one of the few things that *truly* terrified me in the beginning, as I had come to realize that deep down, I had a fear of water and of drowning in it. I was never really a "swimmer" growing up. I was typically comfortable in the water, spent much time playing in pools and lakes and could certainly keep afloat easily enough... but it wasn't until I reached my mid-20s, when I decided I wanted to do a short triathlon, that I quickly realized that what I considered "swimming" wasn't much more than doggy paddling and treading water. I was quickly humbled by my first few attempts at lap swimming. I considered myself a pretty fit individual. I had competed in bodybuilding, and once I gave that up, I continued to work out consistently through weight training, running and biking. Let me tell you what, I thought I was going to DIE swimming one mere lap of the pool. I tried with all my might, but my legs sank, I got a bunch of water in my nose and mouth and I was so winded after attempting to swim 50 yards (2 lengths of the pool)! I was really shocked at how inept I was at lap swimming. This didn't derail me, though. Something else I started to find out in my mid-20s (besides not being able to swim!): I am stubborn and independent, I love a challenge, and I especially don't like obstacles that stand in the way of goals that I want to achieve. If you tell me you think I can't do something, it makes me even more determined to prove you wrong. I don't know where this tenacity came from, but it continues to burn far into my 40s and I love it. So at that time, I became obsessed with improving my swimming technique and fitness, and I devoured every piece of information I could find online, read a book, bought some swim training aids and set to improving my swimming! My goal was to complete my first sprint distance triathlon, which consisted of 800 yards of swimming, followed by 14 miles on bike, followed by a 3 mile run. 800 yards is the equivalent to 16 laps (or 32 lengths) in a standard 25 yard lap pool... that seemed pretty daunting, considering that I felt like one single lap was difficult, but I persisted and I made it to the finish line at my very first sprint triathlon. Although that was about 13 years ago and my memory is a bit fuzzy, I remember two very distinct experiences from my first race: 1. the swim was very hard. I fought through open water anxiety and I came in from the swim feeling wiped and exhausted. I persevered through the bike, which was difficult because I rode an old, used mountain bike and my chain fell off. I have no memories of the run, but I remember #2: the pure feeling of elation that occurred when I crossed the finish line. That very feeling is what hooked me, and why I have done so many more triathlons since! But I digress....

I put quite a bit of work in to get from swimming very little to being able to complete the 800 yards of that first triathlon, which incidentally, is under a half of a mile. I worked to improve my stroke. I swam the necessary training distances in the pool. I got a wetsuit because it helps you float and almost every triathlete wears one. I lined up with the other athletes to begin my swim and I waited for many of them to start before I dove in the water to start the swim. I had read stories about people being punched and kicked and swum over during the beginning of the race and there was no way I wanted anything to do with that, so I started off behind the pack. I started swimming the freestyle stroke I had been working on, aka the old school "crawl" - the stroke used by distance swimmers for its speed and efficiency. I had a really hard time keeping my breathing under control due to the adrenaline-rush of beginning the race, not knowing how to correctly pace myself and still being a long way from what I would consider an "efficient" swimmer. Plus, I am competitive by nature and being passed by other swimmers ramped up my anxiety even more. I was winded, my heart started pounding and I had my very first open water panic attack. Ugh. As I always do when I feel panic coming on in the water, I looked up to see where the nearest kayaker was. Close by, thankfully. Luckily, I was wearing a wetsuit which increases buoyancy, so I wasn't worried about drowning. I was completely overwhelmed and afraid that I wouldn't be able to get through the swim, and for me, not completing something I set out to do is devastating. These thoughts only served to feed my panic and anxiety. I knew I had to suck it up. After all, "Grit" is my middle name (not really!). I rolled onto my back in the water to get control of my breathing. This wasn't my first go-around with battling panic attacks; it was just the first time it ever happened in the water. I took some deep breaths through my nose, gave myself a mini pep talk and then rolled back over to start swimming again. I had to alternate between my version of breaststroke, doggy paddle, backstroke and freestyle. I was not able to keep my breathing controlled enough to swim freestyle the whole way, or even most of the way, from my recollection. But I made it around the buoys and to the swim finish line. Winded and wiped out, I made it out of the water and into the transition area. The whole ordeal took all of about 30 minutes. It was THE longest 30 minutes of my life. I realized that I was not at all a good swimmer, despite the work I had put into it. I made it to the race finish line rather uneventfully, with the exception of dropping a chain during the bike portion. I was elated! I had completed my very first sprint distance triathlon. However, like many other triathletes, I decided that I despised the swim portion of the race. It was difficult and anxiety inducing, and I was just "not a good swimmer."

I completed a few more short triathlons over the years with the same-ish result. I would follow the training plan and complete the suggested workouts for the event that I wanted to participate in. I was always fairly pleased with my performance on the bike and on the run as compared to other participants. I'm not speedy, by any means, and I don't place, but I'd typically have a pretty solid finish. However, the swim portion of the race continued to induce panic and anxiety, and I would still get out of the water feeling like I'd expended an awful lot of energy to swim a fairly short distance. I took a break in racing for a few years as life shifted and my priorities changed, but I came back again.. I always seem to find my way back. Triathlons are what I love to do. I decided to head back to the pool sometime around the beginning of 2016 to pick lap swimming back up again. I had been doing a lot of running races and knew swimming would be a great offset to all the pounding from running. Plus, I had been considering getting back into doing triathlons again. I made a plan to swim twice a week and work on my swim fitness, and I was pretty consistent with that. I went to the pool, I swam my designated number of laps and then I got out. I signed up for another sprint triathlon with my husband and some friends for the summer of 2016. By the time I got to the race, I felt very prepared for the swim since I had been swimming pretty consistently for over 6 months. I was so confident in my swim training that I decided to start with the front of the pack for a change (instead of hanging back), and I also decided to skip wearing the wetsuit since it was hot and the distance was short. The race started and I dove in the water and started swimming. The race went exactly the same as my very first race, only this time my panic was even worse. I looked up to see where the nearest support person was and I couldn't see one because the race was smaller and didn't have as many people on the water as I was used to. And I couldn't rely on the buoyancy of my wetsuit, because I didn't wear one. The body of water at the race location was almost black, and I could see nothing. I had the worst open water panic attack that I had ever had previously, and it was a bit harder to talk myself through this one. I had to work to calm down and bring my heart rate down so I could finish the swim portion of the race, and the swim portion was only about a *quarter* mile.. one of the shortest ones I had completed. I did finish, as I usually do, and I still finished well. But I was so, so discouraged. I felt like for all the time that I had put into swimming, I never got any better at it. I'm quite sure that isn't true. Physically, my swim fitness had certainly improved, but this mental thing, this panic and anxiety, were so scary, and THAT part obviously didn't improve at all. In fact, it seemed even worse on this particular day. I knew that if I couldn't get past that, I would not be able to become a better open water swimmer. I kept swimming in the pool after that but I KNEW I had to do something different if I wanted to do a longer distance triathlon, which was something I REALLY wanted to do. So in December of 2016, I signed up for a two-week trial with the local Masters swim club.

I was certainly intimidated by the prospect of joining a group of people who I did not know and who were, most certainly, much better swimmers than I thought I could ever be, but I knew that if I wanted the outcome of my open water swims to be different, then I had to *change* what I was doing. I had to challenge the boundaries of my "bubble", and see if it was actually possible for me to become a better swimmer. I had my sights set on a half Ironman distance triathlon and I WANTED to be a stronger and more confident swimmer. I was nervous when I showed up at that first practice, but that didn't last long at all. The coaches and club members were extremely welcoming, and I soon realized the club contained members of varying abilities. I started off by going to the less attended practices while my coaches worked with me on improving my swimming form and fitness. I made an effort to attend practice two times a week, and set a goal to swim at least 2000 yards at each practice. I got better and better. Practices became less strenuous for me and I started feeling more energized and less wiped out after each session. At one point, I decided to attend one of the harder practices, the ones that fastest swimmers in the club would attend. That definitely dialed things up a notch. I found myself more winded and more tired after those practices, but I knew that meant I worked harder and that was a good thing! That meant I was getting better.

In June of 2017, I completed my first half Ironman distance triathlon. I swam 1.2 miles in Jamesville Reservoir in Syracuse, New York. That day, the water was a bit choppier than I had anticipated - it is a reservoir, it wasn't supposed to be choppy AT ALL, but that didn't bother me. I got into the water and still hung back some at the start, but I started swimming and I just kept going. No panic, no racing heart, no feeling winded. I was able to swim freestyle the whole way, and when I got out the water, I was absolutely *elated* to find that I felt like I could have kept swimming. I wasn't tired AT ALL. I was excited and energized to continue the race. A year later, I completed my second half Ironman distance triathlon with a better time than the previous year, and in January of 2018, I took the leap and signed myself up for my full distance Ironman race. During that time, I continued swimming with the Masters'

Swim Club and I even started attending more open water swimming events and made new friends with people who were (and still are) better swimmers than I, and who encourage me to continue to step outside my swimming comfort zone. I have swum longer distances and in water conditions that I would likely not have done if it weren't for the support of my swim friends. These experiences are the reason that my open water anxiety has about disappeared: my skill, confidence and swimming fitness level have all grown, and all because I took the leap and joined the club. I did, in fact, become a better swimmer, found a new passion and met new friends who also share the same passion! To date, my longest swim distance is 2.4 miles: the distance of the swim portion of the full distance Ironman, but I intend to join some of my teammates on some longer distances. Not only did I become a better swimmer, but I also found that I absolutely LOVE swimming, now that I am decent at it. It is now my favorite form of exercise, and has enriched my life in ways that I could never have imagined.

So the moral of my very long winded story is that I honestly could have just declared that I was "not a good swimmer" and given up on my hopes to be a better one. But I didn't, even though swimming was really scary for me at times. I pushed past my comfort zone and found that there was a whole new area of my life and the world in which I get to explore with new friends.

Between our expectations and our comfort zones, we find ourselves trapped in the same boring ol' patterns of wishing and wanting and not acting on it, then engaging in the same ol' bad habits and then beating ourselves up over all of it. All you need to do is just make that decision that you are going to do something new. Make a plan. Then follow through and act on it. If you feel afraid or anxious, that's OK. You just need to breathe and do it anyways. "Brave" people are not without fear; they feel fear and they act ANYWAYS. That is the difference.

You will find that as soon as you make that decision, you will feel differently and that as soon as you begin to act on your decision, that things will begin to shift for you.

Maybe you are truly happy staying in your comfort zone all day every day, and you never wish or want for something else or for anything to be different!

In that case, maybe I could have told you paragraphs ago that you could skip to the next section. Oops... For the rest of us, we do *deeply* crave change.. and are just too afraid to actually go after it.

So I pose this challenge to you: Once a day for the next 30 days, do something you have never done before. It could be big or small. Go to a new class, go to a new store, try a new food, take a new way home, say "hi" to a stranger if you don't normally talk to people you don't know.... there are so many options. It's up to you what you choose.

Prioritizing Self Care

"You yourself,
as much as anybody in the entire universe,
deserve your love and affection."
-Sharon Salzberg

I f I had a dollar for every time I heard "I don't have enough time...." from family, friends and patients when it came to fitting in self care appointments.... I'd have a lot of dollars! It makes me crazy! And the worst part? I am totally guilty of putting off my own needed appointments for the sake of time!! What is wrong with us?? Why don't we prioritize our own self care? We manage a million things and take care of others and feel like the things we do are oh, so important! (And they are!) But if we are not well or we are injured or in pain, then we certainly aren't going to be helping others.. and continuing to drain ourselves without refilling our tanks is only going to serve to make us unwell in the future. So doesn't it make sense to make sure that we are in tip-top condition so that we are able to do as much for others as we want to? That MEANS that we should take the time out of our busy lives to make sure we are maintaining our ability to keep moving at light speed.

When I think about this concept, I am reminded of a patient of mine. She is 72 years old and she suffers from pain, weakness and balance issues in her legs and feet. This patient's condition is not something that happened overnight given the visible deterioration of muscle mass in her legs; it was a slow progression that continued over time until one day the patient had decided that it was beginning to interfere with the activities she wanted to engage in, and only then did she seek treatment. Then immediately, she wanted to be better and seemed to be a bit frustrated when her strength hadn't returned after 3 weeks of acupuncture and physical therapy. In order for this patient to regain strength, she has to build her muscle mass back to a functional level, and at 72 years old, that is no quick and easy task. Months to years of deterioration simply can't be reversed in only a few weeks, and the older a person gets, the longer the body takes to bounce back. When presented with the work that was going to be required to improve her condition, this patient would insist that she is "too busy" and that she didn't have "time" to do the exercises and fit in the acupuncture and physical therapy treatments between her zumba and folk dancing classes, horseback riding and volunteer work at the library and animal shelter. What does one say to that? I had to explain to her that her issues didn't happen overnight and that it was going to take a little time and commitment to get back on track, but really.. what choice does one have at that point? Make time or continue to fall apart? Trust me, ignoring your issues will only serve to allow them to get worse and harder to recover from. Ignoring them is foolish.

This concept of "not having enough time" is another wall created by our own minds. We ALWAYS have time. It is just how we prioritize it and the way we choose to use it. If you think that cleaning your kitchen is more important than doing a workout, then you'll choose to clean your kitchen and then declare that you "didn't have time" to work out. Or maybe you chose to sleep over getting a morning run in, or going grocery shopping instead of getting a massage because you "need" groceries, but not a massage. Even a job with long hours is still a choice. It may be a BIG choice to change it, but it is still, in fact, a choice. One of the beauties of living in America is that we are always surrounded by an abundance of choices. Too many, I think sometimes! I used to use the "I don't have time" excuse, but then once I realized that it isn't about *having* the time as much as it is about *making* the time, I started to rephrase it into: "I didn't *make* the time", or "I chose to spend my time doing [x] instead of [y]." It's amazing what you can make the time for if you really want to. I didn't think I had *time* to train for an Ironman, but somehow I managed to free up 3 to 6 hours a day to train. I chose training over sleep, over cooking, over spending time with my husband, my daughter, my dogs, my friends & family and engaging in other activities that I might normally have taken part in on evenings and weekends. I shortened my hours at work. I made it work because it was something I really wanted to do.

It is VERY important that you put effort into maintaining your body and mind, and that you *make* time to do it regularly. These are things you need to do EVERY SINGLE DAY, as maintenance. Exercise is really important, but so is stillness and quiet time and time in places and with people who make you feel happy and content. Time to make sure that you feel comfortable in your own skin. Everyone has their own needs, but we ALL need to put time in the only body that we get to live in for the rest of our lives. Invest in yourself first. And then the super awesome you can spread around your awesomeness to everyone else!

II

The Physical Needs of Women

Two Hundred Thousand Years

elieve it or not, and contrary to what our medical culture in the US portrays, the human body is *extremely* resilient and not nearly as fragile as we are led to believe. Think about this for a second: Human beings have been on this earth for over 200,000 years!! TWO HUNDRED THOUSAND YEARS. So for all that time, humans have lived and reproduced into the population that is on earth today. Does that seem like the human body is fragile and has trouble surviving without the use of modern medicine? "Modern medicine or medicine as we know it, started to emerge after the Industrial Revolution in the 18th century. At this time, there was rapid growth in economic activity in Western Europe and the Americas." (MNT Editorial Team: Medical News Today, 2018). So, medicine as we know it in this country has been around a relatively short period of time in relation to how long humans have been on this planet. A fear has been created in us, however, a fear that we will all perish without the modern technologies of the food and drug industry. This fear, in most cases, has been driven primarily by capitalism, and has resulted in most Americans chronically using prescription and over-the-counter medications, and eating foods created in factories and not in nature. Our modern lifestyles are actually doing just the opposite of what these companies are promising: we are getting sicker and not healthier.

Our medical system focusses on the treatment and alleviation of immediate (acute) symptoms and doesn't spend much time looking at the long term prospects or effects of certain therapies. As a result, our illnesses are showing up in the form of more chronic, more serious illness, like cancer and autoimmune dysfunction. We are definitely keeping people alive in the short term, but what are the long term implications of using medications that mask symptoms and change the normal functioning of the body? And, instead of looking at uncomfortable digestive, menstrual, immune-related and mental/emotional issues as a sign that we need to make changes, we are given medications to alleviate symptoms and not encouraged to make necessary changes, changes that need to be made for *long term* health reasons, thus continuing to live in a state of imbalance.

The body can and will take *years* of constant abuse. We are not as fragile as we are made to believe, and our bodies actually function better and are healthier when we are not constantly dumping harmful chemicals into them. Since our bodies are living materials from this earth, we are meant to consume and be around other living materials from this earth. That is how we will thrive. That is how we can make sure that are bodies are properly nourished. Most of us do not need drugs and other chemicals to be and to stay alive. I do realize that some of us do, but that is the exception, and also possibly a matter of opinion. In many cases, making necessary diet, lifestyle and mental health changes can help to reduce our perceived dependence on chemicals (foods, alcohol, drugs, etc). Moving on....

A Woman's Dietary Needs

So let's talk about physical needs for a bit and things that you CAN do to make improvements. Your diet is the SINGLE most important thing that you maintain on a regular basis that affects your health, and your body's ability to heal itself. **I cannot even begin to tell you how important it is**. It affects EVERYTHING. If you are not taking in what your body needs, your body cannot do any of the million tasks it does on a given day properly. It *especially* cannot heal from damage, whether it is intentional or not. Many of the constituents that our bodies require to build new bones, tissues and blood comes from what we get in our food (and our environment!). Is it possible to repair a wall without proper building materials? Maybe, but what kind of repair will it be? And is that the kind of workmanship that you want holding together the body you need to live in for the rest of your life? You don't! That's because these are the areas that will break down and cause problems later on down the line. Trust me. Being in the healthcare field and seeing people in chronic pain because their bodies never healed well is extremely common. I watch people suffer all the time for reasons that could have been prevented had they just known how. Your body will be able to function and recover much more effectively if you give it the tools it needs to rebuild itself! Our bodies are highly resilient and they are constantly changing over and making new tissues. The body can withstand substantial abuse and heal, but without the proper building blocks, this process is impossible. Prolonged abuse without the ability to heal leads to breakdown, slowly but surely, and eventually, to complete failure.

I know how bombarded we are with information about what we "should" eat. It is so overwhelming for people that they don't even know where to start when it comes to "eating healthy". By now, that term is so overused that I see people's eyes glaze over at the mere use of the phrase. Let me tell you this: I like to keep it simple, and again, operate from my training in Chinese medicine: "everything in moderation." I'll start by saying that I do not believe in eliminating entire food groups, so I am not going to advocate for anything like the "keto" diet or even a vegetarian or vegan diet. I do, however, abide by a few simple rules when it comes to my idea of "eating healthy":

Rule #1: Consume foods that come from the Earth.

Remember that we are beings of planet Earth, and just like every other living being that lives on this planet, we were MEANT to consume foods that are created by this planet, NOT in a factory or a lab by other human beings. I know that as human beings, we like to think that we have it all figured out scientifically and that we know better than mother nature. WE DO NOT. We need foods from the Earth because they contain matter that is *essential* to the proper functioning of our bodies. And contrary to popular scientific opinion, we do **not** know every molecular constituent of food and what it does in our body. We need foods in ways that science has not even yet discovered. So what does this mean? This means that the BEST foods for us to eat are those that come directly from the Earth: fruits, vegetables, nuts, seeds, minimally processed grains, and yes, even meat and animal products. My professional training and experience has shown me that humans do, in fact, need animal protein to operate optimally. I will cover this in a different section.

Now I do understand that in this day and age, most of our foods are processed in some way, shape or form. Very few of us go out and harvest our foods and eat it directly from its growing state. Such is the nature of our world now. Even supermarket fruits and veggies are sprayed with pesticides, picked before they are ripe, packaged, shipped and in some way "processed." In my opinion, it's best to get your food locally if possible from farmers' markets and local shops but this isn't always a possibility. Many of the grain products we consume are highly processed, such as breads, pastas, wraps, rice and other grains. I recommend choosing ones that are as minimally processed as possible. Read your labels! Keep in mind that if it's white, it's probably been bleached and therefore, stripped of nutrients. Not too many foods that are bright white exist in nature. In many cases, processed grains like breads, pastas and cereals are "enriched" with vitamins, meaning they are so stripped of nutrients and the manufacturers add vitamins back into the food after processing. I try to steer clear of these foods, as I liken them to edible cardboard. In my ideal world, my daughter and I would eat nothing out of a package or that I hadn't prepared myself... but what a laughable prospect that is! That would mean I would never have a social meal with anyone that I hadn't prepared myself, that I would be 100% responsible for preparing every single one of my meals for the rest of my life, and that I would likely have to quit doing at least 75% of the activities I love to do so I could spend a majority of my time and effort shopping at multiple places, planning meals, cutting fruits & vegetables (a job I despise for some reason!), cooking, cleaning up and eating. Obviously, it's quite an undertaking! Convenience is certainly important, and much of the social aspect of our culture involves the act of putting food and drink into our bodies. So once again, I reiterate: moderation. We can't be perfect, but you know what we can do? *We can do the absolute best we can do, and nothing more.* A little bit here and there is perfectly fine. Make choices, and choose wisely.

This also leads me to the topic of vitamins and supplements; a topic in which I have mixed feelings about. I do wholeheartedly believe that supplementation in some cases is helpful - I do practice Chinese herbal medicine prescribing, so I do sometimes recommend certain supplements, but I also feel that vitamins and supplements should NOT replace food. I feel that one should eat as healthfully as possible FIRST, and then supplement second. Vitamins and minerals are meant to be extracted from a whole food, and not taken in a pill. There's no way to know if your body even utilizes the pill form of many vitamins. Moreover, many vitamins, minerals and even herbs work in conjunction with one another. For example, there are *eight* B vitamins, and in order to absorb and do what they need to do in the body, there needs to be a certain ratio of each because they work together. So in many cases, it's practically useless to take them in isolation, yet so many people are still doing this because they just don't know. I recommend finding a reputable manufacturer of multivitamins and taking a daily dose, and don't self prescribe based on internet information. It is far too complicated, so if you want to take supplements, you should find someone who is educated on the topic and get recommendations. I have a doctorate and I still find the information confusing and overwhelming. I can't even imagine what it's like for the "layperson."

I recommend eating a "plant-based" diet, and by using the term "plant-based" I mean to eat *mostly* plants. This does not mean you have to eat *solely* plants. I am a big advocate for eating animal products and I will explain why in a few more pages. I believe that *most* of your diet should be made up of fruits, vegetables, whole grains, nuts and seeds. The rest: animal protein sources, such as eggs, some dairy and good quality lean meats and fish, organic if you can get that.

Rule #2: Make your meals as colorful as possible (and not artificially).

The foods that provide the best bang for their nutritional "buck" are fruits and vegetables, and that is because they contain the highest amount of vitamins and phytonutrients. Studies show that people who eat more plant foods have reduced risk of chronic diseases such as diabetes, heart disease, and cancer. Believe it or not, different colored fruits and vegetables contain slightly different nutrient profiles. Refer to the following phytonutrient table to help visualize why eating colorful meals is important for health and wellness.

Color	Phytonutrient(s)	Fruits/Veggies	Main Vitamins
Red	Lycopene	tomatoes & tomato products, red peppers, red cabbage, pink grapefruit, watermelon	Vitamin C, potassium
Red/Purple	Anthocyanins	red grapes, blueberries, blackberries, raspberries, cherries, plums, prunes, red beets, strawberries, red apples, cranberries	Vitamin C, potassium
Orange	Alpha and Beta Carotene	apricots, acorn & winter squash, butternut & yellow squash, carrots, mangoes, cantaloupes, pumpkin, sweet potatoes	Vitamin A, beta carotene, vitamin C, magnesium, potassium
Orange/Yellow	Beta Cryptothanxin	clementines, mandarin oranges, oranges, peaches, pineapples, nectarines, papaya, tangerines, lemons & limes	Vitamin C, folate, potassium
Yellow/Green	Lutein and zeaxanthin	collard greens, green & yellow bell peppers, green beans, kale, mustard & beet greens, spinach, green peas, avocados, honeydew melon, yellow corn	Vitamin C, vitamin K, calcium, folate
Green	Sulforaphane, isothiocyanate and indoles	broccoli & broccoli sprouts, bok choy, brussel sprouts, cabbages, kale, cauliflower	Vitamin C, folate, potassium
White/Green	Allicin and flavonoids	asparagus, celery, chives, endive, garlic, leeks, mushrooms, pearl onions, onions, pears, shallots, artichokes	Selenium, folate

Table 1: Food colors, phytonutrients & vitamins

Let's just review the common phytonutrients for a minute so we can see why eating a variety of colors is important.

Lycopene. Lycopene is an antioxidant and natural pigment that gives some foods (like tomatoes, red peppers, pink grapefruit, watermelon and papaya) their red color. Some studies have shown that lycopene decreases the risk of some cancers, such as breast and prostate cancer, improves cardiovascular health, protects the skin from sun damage, and can improve brain health and eyesight. The largest source of lycopenes in the American diet is clearly tomatoes and tomato products. Sauces and condensed forms of tomatoes are fine in moderation, but may be too acidic for some people. Eating the whole food is always better. (This is why I am not a fan of juices, either. We are not meant to consume such concentrated forms of certain fruits and veggies.)

Anthocyanins. Anthocyanins are in fruits and vegetables and are responsible for the colors, red, purple, and blue. "Anthocyanins possess antidiabetic, anticancer, anti-inflammatory, antimicrobial, and anti-obesity effects, as well as prevention of cardiovascular diseases (CVDs)" (He K, Li X, Chen X, et al.). Anthocyanins are found in dark red & purple colored fruits and vegetables, such as beets, cranberries, blueberries, cherries and blackberries. A popular

Chinese herb found in many Chinese herbal formulas is mulberry, a small purple-black fruit found growing wild in many places in the US. Mulberries are also high in anthocyanins.

Alpha and Beta Carotenes. Alpha and Beta Carotenes are part of the carotenoid family, and are pigments that cause foods to be orange or yellow in color. Alpha and beta carotene are converted to vitamin A in the body and are therefore important precursors. Vitamin A is essential for growth, reproduction, immune function and skin and eye health. Foods that are dark orange in color will fall into this group. Carrots, apricots, mangoes, sweet potatoes and winter squashes are going to be your best sources of alpha and beta carotenes.

Beta Cryptothanxin. Beta Cryptothanxin is very similar to beta carotene. It is another carotenoid that is converted into vitamin A in the body. These foods are a bit lighter in color; they include lighter orange and yellow fruits and vegetables, such as oranges, peaches, lemons, pineapple and yellow peppers.

Lutein and zeaxanthin. Lutein and zeaxanthin are the predominant carotenoids which accumulate in the retina of the eye. "They are the major constituents of macular pigment, a compound concentrated in the macula region of the retina that is responsible for fine-feature vision." (Eisenhauer, 2017). By the way, macular degeneration is the most common cause of blindness in older adults. Foods highest in these phytonutrients are green and yellow in color. Fruits and vegetables such as spinach, green and yellow bell peppers, kale, avocados and corn, and even egg yolks are great sources of lutein and zeaxanthin. So eat your fruits, veggies and eggs if you want to keep your eyesight!

Sulforaphane, isothiocyanate and indoles. This group is found mostly in your family of cruciferous vegetables: broccoli, kale, cabbage, brussel sprouts and cauliflower. This group has powerful anti-inflammatory and anti-carcinogenic capabilities and targeted therapies using concentrated versions of these phytonutrients have been used in the prevention of certain types of cancers. Sulforaphane has been shown to actually INHIBIT proliferation of both prostate and breast cancers, and reverse inflammation in the lungs. In my opinion, foods from this group should be consumed daily! There is a reason why many foods in this group are called "superfoods."

Allicin and flavonoids. Allicin is found in garlic and contains very powerful antibacterial and antiviral, as do most of the "pungent" vegetables and spices, like onions, leeks, and chives. If you want to stay cold and flu-free, add lots of garlic, onion and pungent spices to your diet.

While it is important to make sure you are getting as many phytonutrients as possible, let's pay special attention to **anthocyanins** (also known as anthocyanidins) for a minute. This family of phytonutrients are colored, water-soluble pigments that make up the colors red, purple, and blue in fruits and vegetables. The reason I find this group the most interesting is because in Chinese medicine theory, it is this group of foods that we refer to as "blood building," meaning foods that most resemble the color of blood are those that aid in the production of good quality blood and fluids. Because women menstruate regularly, their bodies are constantly producing new blood, and in pregnancy, they are building blood and tissues in another human being. With that in mind, it is especially important for women to consume foods that help them build and maintain quality blood.

Please note that just because we are looking at these nutrients and foods individually does NOT mean you should take any of these nutrients in isolation. Food vitamins and nutrients are meant to be consumed IN WHOLE, in a combination with other foods, *in moderation*. The body operates through very complex pathways, and if you've ever in your life had to study the Kreb's Cycle, this becomes clear. Many chemicals and nutrients need to work in conjunction with one another in order to get the job done. Let's take a simple example, like building a brick wall. In order to build a brick wall, you need bricks and mortar, right? And tools? And in the right ratio, right? You can't build a brick wall without mortar or bricks (or tools), and if you have too many bricks and not enough mortar, you can maybe build half the wall. The same applies with too much mortar and not enough bricks. You need to have to have all necessary pieces AND in the right ratio, or you can't complete the process. The same applies to our bodies. You only need small amounts of certain nutrients; many chemicals can actually go from being *beneficial* to being *poisonous* simply by the consumed dosage. More does not always mean *better*. This is a common misconception in today's nutritional culture, and I see people supplementing individually with this and that without consult. This is a waste of your time and your money, and could potentially be harmful. Consuming food is fine, as you are unlikely to get too many vitamins/phytonutrients from food... our bodies know how to dump the extra.. but taking extra supplements can get a bit tricky.

What about vitamins? I don't know if this is obvious by looking at the chart, but the biggest problem with substituting manufactured vitamins with food is that you are skipping the nutritional value of the foods: the calories and the phytonutrients. You should aim to get most of your vitamins through food sources, and not expect vitamins and supplements to be an adequate substitute. They are not. All food elements need to be present and work together to promote healing and wellness. With that said, there are a few dietary supplements that I DO recommend be taken regularly.

Green powders: green powders, or "superfood" powders are basically fruits and vegetables that are concentrated into a powder that can be added to smoothies or protein shakes. I feel it is impossible for most people to eat enough vegetables on a daily basis, and while you don't get the fiber and whole food with a powder, you do get all the amazing phytonutrients that I mentioned earlier. I also want to reiterate that because this also not a whole food, this should be used *in addition to*, and *not instead of,* whole foods. I make a protein shake almost every day with a scoop of green powder. The taste does take some getting used to. I'm so used to it that I don't even notice it.. but if someone in my family decides to take a sip of my protein shake, they will remind me that it does taste exactly like what it is... powdered vegetables! A scoop of green powder daily is all you need to really boost your health.

Tart cherry juice: Tart cherries are especially good for women, and wouldn't you know? They are also a naturally occurring source of melatonin. Melatonin is a hormone that your brain produces to help regulate your sleep cycle. In terms of Chinese medicine, tart cherries help to build what we call "yin." As the opposite of "yang," "yin" is the necessary fluids that your body needs to function properly: the plasma in your blood, the mucus produced by your immune, digestive and reproductive systems that help to protect and move things around, the fluid in your joints that keep them moving smoothly and fluidly. Once women approach menopause, common complaints are sleep issues and dryness (dry eyes, dry vaginal fluids, dry stools, etc.) Tart cherries help to moisten the body and held to offset the internal dryness that may set in as a result of hormone imbalance. Tart cherries come in a concentrate or a juice form. You can drink a cup of juice a day or you can use the concentrate in smoothies, protein shakes, in greek yogurt (great bedtime snack!), or in any other way your creative self can come up with.

Herbal supplements: Herbal supplements can be a great addition to a healthy diet, but the caveat here is that you REALLY need to find a practitioner who is trained to prescribe them. I cannot emphasize this enough!!! As a Doctor of Chinese medicine, I have *extensive* training in herbal medicine, including herb-drug interactions. More so than anyone I know that practices in other specialties. The landscape of herbal medicine is very complicated, and it is VERY different from the way pharmaceuticals are prescribed. There are thousands of herbs, and what is appropriate for one patient may not at all be appropriate for another. And make no mistake, just because herbs are considered "more natural" does not mean that they cannot be inappropriately taken or don't have interactions with medications, because they often are and do. So while they are a fantastic tool when used properly, I urge much caution when delving into their use. Please do not just willy nilly pull something off a shelf or use it because it works for your neighbor or sister-in-law. This is not a good idea. I am guilty of this myself before I went to school for Chinese medicine, where I then learned how complex herbal medicine really is. Now I emphatically advise against it. With the training I have, I can use herbal medicine to effectively treat almost any ailment that afflicts myself, my family and my patients. I was able to avoid giving my daughter any antibiotics until she was 11 years old by simply treating her childhood illnesses with Chinese herbs. People around me will ask for certain formulas by name because they know Chinese herbs can treat their issues, often better and without the side effects of pharmaceuticals. Herbal remedies have been around for thousands of years! If you are interested in going this route, my advice is that you find someone trained to administer them in your area. In fact, I recommend it!

Rule #3: Get enough protein.

Quality protein intake is SO, SO important, *especially* for women. Did you know that a woman's body actually has the tendency to catabolize itself (ie. break down its own tissues) during certain parts of the menstrual cycle, during pregnancy and into menopause? Keep in mind that the #1 goal of a woman's body is procreation and her body will, in fact, break down its own tissues in an effort to achieve and sustain a pregnancy, and to produce a new human being... and once that time has passed, the decline in hormone levels again triggers tissue loss. This is the reason women lose muscle mass, bone density and even blood volume after menopause. The best way to combat the loss is to maintain adequate protein intake, as well as to exercise: weight bearing exercise is especially important during this time to maintain muscle mass and bone density. The whole saying "move it or lose it" applies well to the human body. If you are not using every part of your body regularly, it will weaken. Think about what happens to a car when you let it sit and don't run it.. it deteriorates, breaks down JUST FROM SITTING THERE and stops being able to function. The same thing happens to our bodies when we stop challenging them. Tissues that require a lot of bodily energy to maintain, such as skeletal muscle, will not be maintained by the body if they are not being used. Why would it? Would you want to continue to maintain that car you don't drive?

I have been obsessed with my protein intake since the days when I started bodybuilding in my 20s and I have been carrying my own lunch cooler around with me since then. Yes, for 20 years, I have been toting a lunch cooler back and forth to work.. I have endured my share of jokes at my expense, but that never fazed me. Nutrition has always been a high priority for me, as I have believed for many years that food is medicine. It is common knowledge in the world of sports nutrition that protein is required to build and repair muscle mass, but what is less talked about is that it is *also* required to maintain organ and bone health, and to build and maintain adequate blood volume. Remember that our bodies are organisms that are **constantly** building, repairing and regenerating. Therefore, we NEED an adequate supply of building blocks (one major building block is protein), to assure that our bones, blood and soft tissues are as strong and healthy as we need them to be. Current dietary recommendations such as the infamous **RDA** (Recommended Dietary Allowance) were put in place many years ago to set numerical guidelines for the purpose of preventing malnutrition. Therefore, these numbers represent the *minimum* nutritional requirements needed to keep the average human being alive. ALIVE. Functioning at our most basic level. This is a bare minimum, and these numbers should not be strictly followed by healthy, thriving, active, busy individuals... and depending on body size, type, age and activity levels, you can see that there's no way that one number can fit all. SO. The RDA recommends an absolute **minimum** daily intake of 0.8g of protein per kilogram of body weight. Since most of us Americans don't use kilograms as a weight measurement, I have simplified it into approximately 0.36g of protein per pound of body weight. What this suggests is that 54g of protein per day is the minimum amount required to sustain minimal function of a 150 lb human body. Now I suppose if you laid around in a bubble all day, didn't get much exercise, get sick or injured, this may be enough.. but otherwise, no, this is nowhere near enough protein. 0.8g – 1.0g per pound of body weight is a better number, although keep it mind that it really DOES depend on your lifestyle. If your lifestyle requires that your body undergo frequent repairs due to exercise, injury or illness, then you will have higher protein requirements than others who have different lifestyles. Those who have more muscle mass or who are larger framed will need more protein to maintain the increased size. I firmly believe that women need more than men due to our body's tendency to eat into our existing supply and most DEFINITELY if you are pregnant! And don't forget that if we are not pregnant, we BLEED every single month. So we are constantly building blood also. We are human beings; we are complicated and we don't fit into "one size fits all" plans. But 0.8 - 1g of protein per pound is a good place to start, especially since more women don't consume nearly that much unless they are making the effort. For a 150 lb female, that ends up calculating out to 120 - 150g/day. For reference, a 3oz serving of boneless, skinless chicken breast contains about 28g of protein. So chew on that for a minute!

Let's not forget that humans get many important vitamins and minerals from animal meat sources (protein isn't their only value) such as good fats, vitamin A, K, iron and B12...

Getting enough protein in a day can certainly be a challenge, so it will likely be necessary to supplement with protein powders and protein bars. I find the following sources of protein to be most helpful in my daily life: protein powders & bars (will explain more in a minute), lean meats and fish, eggs, cottage cheese & greek yogurt. Keep in mind that many vegetables, grains, nuts and seeds contain protein, but these sources typically contain lower protein levels, and often don't contain all the essential amino acids that the body needs. It is entirely possible that vegan- and vegetarian diets can contain enough protein, but it requires *education*, *effort* and *planning*. More so than if you are a meat eater! There is a lot of controversy about whether or not humans are meant to eat meat. It is my opinion that they are. This is based on many years of experience, research and in patient care. I still do believe that MOST of our diet should be plant-based, but that we do have protein requirements that should be met to maintain optimal health.

There are certain protein supplements that I recommend. These can be helpful if you are struggling to get enough protein in.

Protein powders/shakes: There is a huge market for protein powders, shakes and bars. This makes it easy to increase your protein. The hardest part is deciding which one to BUY. There are a ton of choices. First you should decide which kind of protein you want. I recommend whey (if you are OK with dairy/animal sources) or rice/pea protein powder if you are not. Whey is one of the most easily digestible forms of protein, but if you have dairy issues, it might not be the best for you. Rice/pea protein powders often have all the essential amino acids added to them to make sure they are balanced. Then I would check labels. I check to make sure the brand includes the amino acid profile. This lists the quantities of each of the nine essential amino acids. It should have AT LEAST 1.2g of L-leucine. The second thing I look for is artificial sweetener. Sucralose hides in many protein powders, and I do not like that. Most protein powders are sweetened to make them more palatable. I prefer more natural sweeteners: fructose, maltodextrin, cane sugar, brown rice syrup, etc. Also, I don't recommend soy protein, unless you can find one that is non-GMO. Unfortunately, most soy is now genetically modified. Last, but certainly not least: I recommend sampling before you commit to buying a large container.. one brand can taste entirely different from another, and some are bad and some are good. You can get creative with protein shakes by adding fruit, fiber supplements, nut butters, green powders, vegetables.. they can be downright tasty!

Protein bars: Protein bars are my go-to for "grab and go," high protein foods. I don't know how people function without them. While I generally prefer minimally-processed (and protein bars are definitely NOT that), sometimes I just just don't have the ability to grab a real meal. If I am going to be on the go a lot on a particular day, I will probably have a protein bar in my purse. These can vary greatly as well, in terms of taste and ingredients. I try to stick with non-GMO ingredients and steer clear of artificial sweeteners. My favorites are the CLIF Builder© bars. I love CLIF© products in general. Great products, great company! Again, don't commit to buying a whole box before you try one. If I am looking for a protein bar, I will look for ones with 20+g of protein. "Energy" bars have around 10g. I use these when hiking or doing other long workouts that require me to eat during. Or I stick to fruit and nut bars - simplest of ingredients - for quick snacks during my workday.

The Protein Controversy

There are certainly varying opinions on how much protein one should eat. I have seen many sources that claim that "Americans eat too much protein." Now, I am now sure who "these" Americans are, but they are NOT the women I see most often coming into my clinic. The women I see are NOT eating enough protein. Not even close. Maybe "these Americans are the "meat and potatoes" eating men of America (the ones eating way too much animal meat and not enough plant-based foods.. but like I said.. after seeing patients for over 10 years, I do NOT agree that "Americans eat too much protein." I think the opposite is true, especially for WOMEN. Women are typically NOT the "meat and potato" people. I also think that Americans tend to not eat enough plant-based foods in general.. eating a variety and the right ratio of foods (moderation!) is extremely important. Let's not JUST blame the protein, people! I have an enormous amount of experience in this area. Not only have I extensively researched this topic over the past 20 years, I am living proof that eating a lot of protein results in being strong, healthy and rarely sick or injured. While I watch my athletic counterparts struggle through injuries that derail their training, I keep training. So you tell me.

Kidneys Vs. Protein

Another blanket myth is that "too much protein damages the kidneys." First of all, this alone is not going to damage your kidneys. IF you end up with kidney problems, it is either because you have a genetic predisposition to it, or there are other issues at play. If it happens to be diet-related (and that is a hard thing to prove), it is likely the result of a poor overall diet for many years. It is true that the kidneys handle the amino acid byproducts of protein breakdown. "The more amino acids that need removing, the harder the kidneys have to work. And for people with kidney disease, this can mean an acceleration of their kidney disease. So if a person stops eating protein, then they are saving their kidneys, right? No, because if we didn't eat protein, then malnutrition would develop and more illness would occur. So the solution is to eat enough protein to maintain health, but to minimize the excess amino acids and spare the kidneys. The way to do this is to eat foods with proteins that cause the least waste, that is, foods that have the right amounts (ratios) of different amino acids that the body will use most efficiently. Since we are animals, foods that come from animals (dairy foods, eggs, meat, poultry, fish) have the best combination of amino acids and produce the least waste- the "high biologic value" or HBV foods." (The Nephron Information Center©, 2004-13) Eggs, by the way, are the PERFECT food when it comes to amino acid ratios. Why wouldn't they be? They have to have everything needed for a tiny new being to develop and grow!

Rule #4: Don't Overeat

This one is really simple. Listen to your bodily cues and stop eating when you are full. Continuing to eat because of old school ideas that you need to "finish your plate," or packing dessert in just because you can is NOT nourishing to your body. Overeating is damaging and overwhelming to the body. Your body lets you know when it is full, so listen. Our bodies only have to ability to process so much food at once. If you are not used to listening to your body, now is a great time to start! It will tell you all you need to know. In addition, don't eat when you are not hungry. Unfortunately, in our culture, this is customary. Pressure to eat at social situations is rampant. Some people even take offense when you don't eat their food at gatherings, and you may even have to deal with some upset folks over the whole business. Some folks were raised to believe that eating is a sign of politeness and not eating is rude. But remember, that is their issue and not yours. Food is fuel for the body. It should not be used for emotional pacification for them or for you and if it is, this may be an area to consider working on. Again, moderation. Overeating will happen. Just be mindful and consider not making a habit of it. Chronic overeating damages the digestive system and causes systemic inflammation, something we call "dampness" in Chinese medicine. Occasional overeating will remind you that it makes your body uncomfortable and so hopefully you'll continue to make it only an "occasional" thing.

Societal pressure to eat and drink really is NO JOKE. This can be really hard to navigate depending on your social circles. When I was in my 20s, I started lifting weights at a local gym and decided that I wanted to try competitive bodybuilding. This is when I officially started toting around my cooler full of food. Most people don't realize just how INTENSE the dieting is that is required for getting body fat levels in women low enough to see the kind of muscle definition one needs to compete in a bodybuilding show. I'm talking MONTHS of strict calorie and macro (carbs, protein, fat) counting and no alcohol, mostly because alcohol lowers inhibition and makes one less likely to stick to the diet plan. An intense diet plus a training plan that included early morning "fasted" cardio sessions to burn more body fat meant that I had ZERO social life. It was then that I fully realized that the culture I grew up and lived in meant that you put calories into your body for *fun*, to be social, to *fit in*, and to avoid snarky comments, odd looks and criticism. Is it any wonder why so many Americans are overweight??? Family and friend gatherings were super stressful because they meant I had no control over what I was served, and avoiding alcohol made them even more awkward. I would often hide protein bars in my purse and occasionally full meals in the cooler in my car, or make sure to eat right before I went. That certainly put some people off and made me look like a crazy person! Most people can't possibly fathom adhering to the dietary lifestyle required to compete in bodybuilding. In fact, many people can't even relate to wanting to eat vegetables and skipping dessert! After 20 years of being a "food snob," I've gotten over caring about offending people by my diet choices. By no means do I diet like I did then – hell no – but I do pick and choose what I will eat and I often come to a party bearing dishes to pass that are loaded with veggies!

And holidays?? UGH. Why is it that holiday traditions consist of gorging oneself until the point of feeling sick? And what "traditional" holiday meal even contains a green vegetable? Is mixing green beans with cream of mushroom soup really the only way you can get someone to tolerate a green vegetable?? But it shows that culturally, we already have a disordered view on eating, and this is what we have to work on undoing if we ever hope to improve the overall health of Americans.

Rule #5: Think of Food as Nourishment. Like Fuel In Your Tank.

FOOD IS FUEL.

That's it. Plain and simple. If you think of food as anything other than that, that is the *first* thing you will need to work on if you want to make dietary changes so that your body is better nourished. Tell yourself (and others!) that you are eating to nourish your body. If the person that you are telling thinks this is funny, then this should just further convince you that culturally, we need to do a better job of making our health a priority. We'd all be a lot better off. Not only would we feel better, but we wouldn't have to pay so much for our healthcare insurance!

Many foods in the American diet are pretty much devoid of positive nutritional value, and are actually harmful instead. Foods deep-fried in really cheap, genetically modified oil? Or meat cooked on a fast food grill that is covered in it?

Desserts? Let's face it.. no one eats dessert because they are actually "hungry." They eat dessert for the sheer enjoyment that some people glean from it. My personal opinion on dessert is that it's a waste of calories. Once in awhile? Sure. Eating dessert every single night? Probably not the best plan. Too much sugar is really problematic and is not going to help your body be more nourished. It's going to detract from it. And this leads to overeating, which we talked about in the previous section!

And yes, you can absolutely enjoy your fuel! There are a MILLION amazing recipes on the internet these days that give you step by step instructions on how to make some pretty healthy, nourishing and flavorful meals (and desserts!) without using a single ingredient that has harmful additives. Take a look. When I am looking for wholesome recipes (specifically ones that don't involve the use "Cream Of" <Whatever> soups), I use the word "paleo" along with whatever I'm searching for. "paleo chili instant pot," "paleo chicken breast recipes," "paleo soup recipes," etc. "Whole30" is another whole foods diet plan that is similar to paleo, so you could use that as a search method too.

Some Thoughts About Mainstream "Diets"

I know a lot of women like the structure of a "diet" plan because it simplifies the complexity of eating, and I also realize that most do it as a means to lose weight. I'm not big into "fad" diets, because most of them eliminate entire food groups that I believe belong in a healthy diet, but there is one "diet" in particular that really resonates with me. The Paleo diet. If you've never heard of it, it is named for the Paleolithic era or "caveman" time, and is a time period where humans were eating only what could be hunted or gathered with no processing of foods. This essentially means that the diet should be made up of meat, fish, fruits, vegetables, nuts and seeds, no grains and no processed foods. Foods straight from the earth with no changing from their original form except for cooking. What I really like about this diet is that it reminds me of how sparse most Americans consumption of vegetables really is. The diet guidelines happen to be very close to my own beliefs on what a quality diet looks like: colorful foods, foods from the earth, and plenty of protein. The best part is that you can eat as much as you want, so if you are a "volume" eater like me, you will be satiated... your tendency to overeat on this diet is rather low because you fill up quickly and there are few foods (if any!) on it that you will be tempted to overeat! I know from the very core of my being that THIS is the way human beings are supposed to eat.

Unfortunately, the odds are stacked against us. Eating this way is a TON of freakin work! I love to eat vegetable packed meals. So much that it makes me giddy! But do I love to prepare vegetables? I don't. I actually despise chopping vegetables, I don't know why. When I eat this way, I spend hours preparing vegetable dishes, like soups, roasted vegetable medleys and salads. I buy a heaping pile and spend a fortune at the grocery store on vegetables, only for them vanish into my belly in under a week. The vegetable part is awesome and I feel so good, physically and mentally, knowing that I am eating amazingly well, but I get burnt out by the meal prep. And quickly. There are so many other things that I would rather be doing than to be stuck in my kitchen cooking. And this is probably the biggest reason that I don't eat this way all the time. And probably a lot of people's reasons for not eating as well as they could. It's expensive and time consuming, and in America, these are typical obstacles.

I often reflect on how terrible the "American" diet really is, and it completely baffles and angers me that we are such a "rich", developed country and our typical dietary staples reflect poverty levels. Most of the foods we consider to be "American:" burgers, french fries, pizza, macaroni & cheese, pasta, macaroni "salad", ice cream... all of these foods are extremely cheap and were created to feed a lot of people very inexpensively. Inexpensive typically means highly processed. They are also devoid of nutrition and possibly even harmful, depending on who you are and where you are getting it. Just recently I was on a road trip to my daughter's lacrosse tournaments and I watched the food signs on the highway as I passed by.. "BURGERS & FRENCH FRIES!", "ICE CREAM", "BEER", "PIZZA". I really want to know: WHY do we continue to eat this way when we are one of the richest countries in the world? Why do we continue to feed our people garbage food?! And not only that... many fast food restaurants provide very few nutritious options for customers who actually care about their nutrition. On this particular road trip, I was determined to continue my "paleo ways" so I brought most of my own food. But I can only get so far with a bag full of "snack" foods. Eventually I need something with more substance. The two times we did stop for food, I ate dry salads as that was the only meat & vegetable option that did not include processed flour products or GMO oils (like those found in most cheap salad dressings that, unfortunately, typically accompany the healthier food options!!) I was actually grateful to at least have that, even though I'm not much of a "salad for a meal" fan... many places don't offer salads at all. On the other hand, a handful of places have more options but my traveling companions were not interested in making nutritious choices (as most people aren't), and so I was outnumbered.

I recognize what a very real challenge it is for busy women to eat well. It also drives home the fact that POOR nutrition is THE BIGGEST cause of sickness and disease in our country. Most Americans are actually undernourished. Yes, they are eating plenty and many are even overweight to prove it. But they are still NOT getting the actual nutrients that their bodies need to achieve and maintain wellness.

We all NEED (like, seriously.. our lives depend on it!) to figure out a way to make time to eat to nourish our bodies. I told my husband that my goal one day is to have a personal chef. Talk about expensive! But hey! My time is worth it, and so is my health.

So I'm gung ho and I eat like a champ for awhile, until I get tired of the meal planning, prep, cooking grind.. life shifts again and then I settle back into eating "pretty well" and into the same old habits. That's just me. I ebb and I flow. And that's OK. I do my best and know that if I wanted to devote my life to being in a kitchen, I would have chosen an entirely different career. I already spend way more time in one than I would like. I get tired of it and frustrated, but eating well is extremely important to me so I suck it up and do what I need to do to maintain that. Where I live, there is no other alternative as local restaurants really do not provide the kind of fare that I consider to be "nutritious." Oh, how I would love to eat perfectly all of the time. It's not possible! So I settle for most of the time. "Bad" foods in moderation, just like everything else!

And speaking of "diets," there is no one "diet" that is appropriate for everyone, as every individual has different needs and dietary sensitivities, due to their genetics, metabolism and lifestyle. I truly wish it were as simple as a "one size fits all" diet that works for everyone across the board. The biggest problem is that it doesn't exist. Women have different needs than men. Adults have different needs than children, who have different needs from elderly. Different body types and ethnicities have different dietary needs depending on their physical origin on this planet. That is because ethnicities developed different survival needs, and therefore different bodily makeup, than others. For example, the dietary needs of Eskimos in Alaska and are going to be entirely different than those from much warmer climates. You will see that the body types between the two are also entirely different, as people from colder climates will tend to be larger and have more of a tendency to retain bodyfat (to keep the warm), than those from warm climates who do not need that. So naturally, each "structured" diet has its own population of naysayers because not every diet works for every person. For example, cutting food groups like dairy and gluten out is absolutely appropriate for some people, but does not work for others. Some people function more optimally on lower carb diets while others cannot function.. and the fasting fad.. oi, there's another one. Great for some, but borderline dangerous for others. Weight loss is a HUGE money making industry, which is why companies are always trying to capitalize on it by trying to provide some "magic pill." THERE IS NO MAGIC PILL. There never has been and there never will be! It frustrates me that the "diets" that get the most attention are typically the ones that are most unhealthy. You have to work on properly *nourishing* your body. Only THEN will you be able to maintain a healthy weight.

So I know what you are thinking now... How do I know what kind of diet is appropriate for me? And that is the million dollar question!

What Kind of "Diet" IS Appropriate For YOU?

There are a lot of things to take into consideration when it comes to your diet. You also have to understand that what works for one person may not necessarily work for you and your lifestyle. Diets are extremely individual. Some people can tolerate some foods while others can't. The goal when selecting a type or types of diet is to choose foods based on their health factor and also on how they make you feel. If you feel terrible after eating certain things, this is your body's way of telling you that that particular type of food isn't for you. Also, many people don't know this, but food sensitivities can show up as non-digestive system related symptoms such as chronic joint pain and post-nasal drip. If you are suffering from chronic issues, consider looking closely at your diet. It is very likely that you could alleviate your symptoms tremendously just by tweaking your diet. Here are the categories I suggest you take a look at:

Dairy

What is so hairy about dairy, anyways? Should you be dairy free? Dairy products give some people a really hard time... and this is why. Think about other species on Earth for a second and tell me.. can you think of one single species, other than humans, in which the individuals 1- drink the milk of another species, and 2- drink milk when they are adults?

Most dairy products that are consumed in this country are from cows, which are a species of animal MUCH larger and MUCH different than humans. Now, I'm not sure if many people realize this, but humans are not cows. I mean, REALLY. They are not!! The composition of cow's milk is actually really **not** appropriate for humans and there is evidence that suggests that humans cannot effectively break down all the components contained in cow's milk. For some people, this shows up very obviously in digestive upset. For other people, the reactions may be a little more subtle. Some people have extremely robust digestive systems and can handle the cow's milk more effectively. (Typically young people, as dairy becomes harder to digest for older people). Common signs that your body is having trouble digesting dairy include increased mucus production after consumption (extra phlegm in the nose and throat, or a feeling of having something stuck in the throat), nausea, stomach pain, bloating, gas, diarrhea. All of these things indicate that your body is creating an inflammatory response to what you are putting in it. For people with chronic allergies, post nasal drip, cough with phlegm in the chest, stomach or intestinal issues or chronic joint pain, I would most definitely recommend a diet of limited dairy. Fortunately, there are also foods that *reduce* mucus, such as lemon, garlic and ginger. This is why it is important that you are eating a good *mix* of different types of natural foods. They will *balance* themselves out.. as long as you are not eating too much. Again... that moderation thing! Small amounts of cheese is fine, but I would advise against drinking *glasses* of milk or other milk-based products, plus eating cheese and yogurt, for example.

Dairy is actually what we consider a "mucus producing" food group, which means it increases the production of phlegm and mucus in the body.

See chart for examples of mucus-producing and mucus eliminating foods.

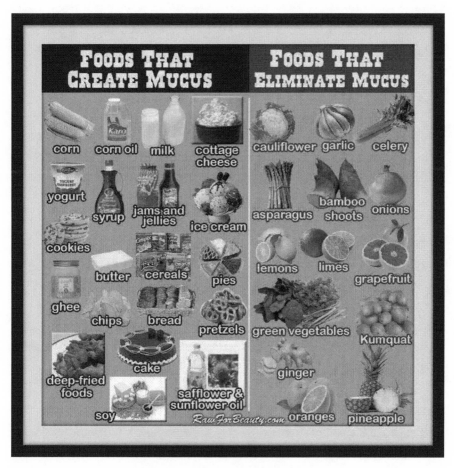

FOODS THAT CREATE MUCUS

corn | corn oil | milk | cottage cheese
yogurt
syrup | jams and jellies | ice cream
cookies
butter | cereals | pies
ghee
chips | bread
pretzels
cake
deep-fried foods
safflower & sunflower oil
soy

FOODS THAT ELIMINATE MUCUS

cauliflower | garlic | celery
asparagus | bamboo shoots | onions
lemons | limes | grapefruit
green vegetables | Kumquat
ginger
oranges | pineapple

Raw For Beauty.com

Photo Credit: RawForBeauty.com

Hard cheeses and yogurt tend to be the easiest of the dairy group to digest as the culturing process helps to assist the digestive process by breaking down some of the molecules. Milk products from smaller animals, like goat milk, tend to be easier for humans to digest. Dairy products increase mucus production in some folks, but not in others, and no one really knows why.

It is likely that genetic predisposition, as well as potential lifestyle factors and even age, dictates one's tolerance to dairy products. With that said, if you find that these symptoms happen to you when you consume dairy, it is best to limit consumption. Chronic inflammation is not something that we want hanging around in our bodies if we can help it. Chronic inflammation is what will result if you continue to consume foods that your body creates this inflammatory response to. Just sayin.

It is recommended that people with chronic phlegm issues, such as sinus issues, post-nasal drip, allergies, asthma, COPD and even joint pain that worsens with damp weather should lean more towards mucus removing, and those without should work towards balancing. If you have ANY issues that worsen when it rains.. guess what? You could benefit from cutting back on mucus-producing foods. Damp external environments will exacerbate damp internal environments. Damp = mucus and phlegm. There is a really easy, Chinese medicine way of finding out just how damp (mucus-y, phlegm-y) you are. Go in your bathroom and take a look at your tongue in the mirror. Does it have a white or yellowish coating on it? How thick or thin is it? Is it in the front or the back or all over? You may brush it off with your toothbrush, which may make it hard to tell. I recommend not doing that for a few days if you are curious. If you have a thicker coating - this is not good - I definitely recommend making some changes. Your diet can and will absolutely change this!

There are MANY milk substitutes these days. I recommend organic coconut milk. Almond milk is becoming quite popular also. Soy milk... eh... not a fan. Unfortunately, most soybeans are genetically modified these days (corn, too!), and since the effects of genetically modified foods on the human body are largely unknown, I personally prefer to stick to foods that are as close to their original source as possible. Using other types of "milk" products will help add more variety to your diet and help to avoid overdoing it. Cow's milk products are extremely prevalent in our culture and in our grocery stores! Maybe some of your favorite foods contain it.. no worries.. just look for places in your diet where you can maybe change it up a bit. Keep your favorite things (like chocolate, maybe? - who's doing away with that?!) and do away with some of the others that you care less about. Unless you are fully lactose-intolerant (in which case, you know what you need to do!), then you do not need to fully cut out all dairy products for the rest of your life. As I mentioned, just think of ways you can cut back.. and occasionally maybe you will overeat it. Oh well. It happens! When it does, your body will likely remind you why you maybe decided to cut back in the first place.

Gluten

Gluten itself is NOT evil, but it does get a bad rap. Gluten is actually a type of protein found in wheat. I've heard people mention the fact that gluten allergies did not exist "way back when," so why are so many people "allergic" to gluten these days? Well, the answer lies not in our own bodies, but in the wheat crops themselves. Modern wheat is not genetically modified, but it is hybridized, which is basically cross-breeding of different varieties for the purpose of increasing yield and disease resistance. "Wheat has been hybridized during the last 50 years to such an extent that it has increased the gluten content exponentially. Not only that, hybridization has created new strains of gluten — one study found 14 new ones." (Edmunds, 2013). It is entirely possible that many people just can't properly digest this "new" wheat, which was changed much more quickly than a usual evolutionary process would take. This "new" wheat was not naturally occurring in nature, and therefore, it may confuse our bodies when attempting to digest it. Who knows! Let's not forget that, collectively, as Americans, we eat way more wheat products on any given day than we should. Bread? Our staples? Pizza, burgers, hot dogs, sandwiches? Pasta/macaroni? Pancakes? Cereal? Cakes, cookies, donuts, muffins? Can you see where I am going with this? Try going to eat out at a local diner when avoiding gluten. Plus many foods have wheat gluten as an additive, such as soy sauce, marinades, dry nuts, and even cosmetics and skin care products. Wheat gluten is used for the purpose of making products a desirable consistency, not for any actual nutritional purpose.

So while you may not necessarily care about how wheat is produced, the take away from this is that wheat IS a problem for many people, and that is why the popularity of "gluten-free" diets are on the rise. I personally find it helpful to *mostly* omit both dairy and gluten.. don't forget about the concept of moderation! You do NOT need to totally omit these things from your diet (unless you have Celiac's disease, in which case - YES, you have to completely omit it.) But this is a special case, and those who suffer from celiac's disease already know what they need to be doing. Take a serious look at how many flour products you are consuming on a daily basis and think about alternatives.

To be completely honest, most flour products, IN GENERAL, are not nutritious, whether they have gluten in them or not. And the amount of preservatives contained in them is, frankly, a little bit scary. Bread that can sit on your counter for a month and not get moldy?? How can that happen?! So turning to a box of gluten free cookies or "gluten-free" pasta made with rice flour is actually NOT a better choice, nutritionally. These products are still highly processed and stripped of essential nutrients during the processing. "Flour" is generally highly processed, as you are taking a full grain and turning it into a powder. Unfortunately, this processing strips the grains of the nutrients that make them so fantastic for you in the first place! Not to mention, these kinds of foods fill you up and take space away from other, much more nutritious foods.. like fruits and vegetables! The foods I specifically mentioned earlier: cereal, bread, pasta, cookies, cakes, donuts, etc, are all very highly processed foods and I recommend trying to limit ALL processed foods, including "gluten-free," "dairy-free," "sugar-free." Just because they are "free" of something, doesn't make them better for you. These foods are nothing but the food manufacturer's way of trying to make a buck on people who don't know any better. Again, fine in moderation.. if you have a hankering for cookies on occasion, go for it... but I would advise against simply replacing your usual flour-based products for the "gluten-free" variety and thinking this is a more nutritious choice. It isn't. Replacing them with more whole food options is your best bet. Being mindful of your choices is really what is important, and making sure that you are eating for the sake of nourishing your body.

About the only processed "bread" product I use regularly is Ezekiel bread, when I am home or can bring my own somewhere. It is one of the most nutritious, minimally-processed breads on the market. In fact, it comes frozen because it isn't loaded with preservatives. Even then, I use it for toast only. It doesn't really make good "sandwich" bread, in my opinion. If I am eating out, I will most often trade wraps for sandwiches to avoid all the bread. Now, let me warn you.. if you are a big regular bread fan and eat it often, there are virtually no good substitutes for it. It is unique and that is why it has such a firm hold in our culture. (Same thing with cheese!) You will likely need to be creative and possibly find new meals that don't involve toast or sandwiches. I typically live on dinner leftovers when it comes to lunches.

Sugar

Oh, the dreaded sugar talk.. I'm pretty sure that by now, most people are well aware of the fact that sugar, in its highly processed forms, is not conducive to bodily health. "Sweet" foods are really not naturally occurring in nature. Suppose we take a look at the "paleo" style diet that I talked about in a previous section. Where in nature do we find "sweet" foods? Fruits, mostly. Some veggies can be on the sweeter side. You can find honey, maple syrup and agave in nature. (Although maple syrup and agave both go through processing to reach the end state that we are used to - they are basically boiled down and concentrated). So you are looking at very *few* naturally-occurring sweeteners. To me, this means that us creatures, living off the earth, are not meant to consume the excess of sweet foods that many do on a daily basis. So, what does "not meant to" mean, in these terms? Our bodies are designed to process certain types of food and because we are creatures of this earth, we are designed with the ability to process foods that come *from the earth*, not from a factory or laboratory. Processing and manufacturing *changes* the composition of our foods and makes our bodies less likely to know how to process them.

It's really not your fault if you have a sugar addiction. As Americans, we have a serious sugar problem. Sugar is like a drug to the human body, and this "drug" drives an entire food and drink industry: soda, candy, cookies and other sweet snacks.. it's a huge industry and the biggest consumers are parents, buying for their children. And this addiction continues for many into adulthood unless someone makes a concerted effort to change it. *Most* Americans, in their transition from childhood to adulthood, have to also transition away from consuming so much sugar for health purposes!

Recently, a friend donated a bunch of baby food to me because my little chihuahua had most of his teeth pulled out and I thought that baby food might be a good option for getting nutritious food into him. What I found was pouch after pouch of sweetened baby food, vegetables hidden in concentrated fruit juice: apple, pear and spinach, apple, banana, and broccoli... hmmmm! Then we wonder why our children won't eat their vegetables. I honestly wouldn't even feed that to my dog! The sweet taste is definitely more palatable for children, and so companies take advantage of that so that children will like their food. We do the same to avoid the frustration of our children refusing food. We are *conditioning* our children to be sugar addicts, and we do it because we think we are *helping* them. We think they might starve otherwise. They won't! And we are actually doing more damage than we are good. Raise your children to eat *real* food, even from infancy, and then they will grow into adolescents and adults that are not afraid of eating green vegetables. If they are *conditioned* to eat vegetables in the same way that they are *conditioned* to eat sugar, we will all be in a lot better shape. And our kids won't have to struggle to "quit" their sugar addiction later in life, like many adults do.

Sugar changes your palate. When you are used to consuming sweet foods, foods that are unsweetened don't taste very appealing to you and it becomes harder to distinguish the more subtle flavors of foods. All you know is that you miss the sweetness. Taking it away can definitely be a bit of an adjustment, but your tastes *do* actually change over time. For example, I mentioned before that I add a super green powder to my daily protein shake. When I first started using the powder, I could taste the "grassy," ground-up-plant flavor. It was slightly unpleasant, but tolerable to me. I am used to more earthy tastes. I have continued to drink the same protein shake almost every day for easily over a year now, maybe more. I don't even taste the green powder anymore. But when someone in my family decides to try my shake, they emphatically let me know how "bad" it tastes. I don't taste it at all... I also don't drink it for the taste.. I drink it because it's *good* for me. Just know that, like the rest of your body, your tastes will ALSO adapt and you will find unsweetened foods more appealing.

Sugar is actually inflammatory. Because it doesn't really belong in the human body, the body often creates an inflammatory response to its presence. What does that mean? That means that high sugar diets can cause weight gain, obesity, chronic pain, fatigue, hormonal imbalances and it has even been linked to encouraging certain cancers to grow within the body. According to the Johns Hopkins School of Medicine, "Cancer cells have been long known to have a 'sweet tooth,' using vast amounts of glucose for energy and for building blocks for cell replication." (John's Hopkins website: Cancer Cells Feed on Sugar-Free Diet). This is where the phrase "sugar feeds cancer" came from, if you've ever heard that. It is true.

Now please don't take this to mean that you're going to get cancer if you eat a few cookies, or a donut. I know that the amount of information in this book is probably overwhelming, but if you take *anything* away from reading this book, I hope it's that you give yourself permission to engage in **moderation**. The health issues I mentioned earlier occur as a result of *chronic overuse.* This means many days, many weeks, many months and possibly many years of consuming too much sugar will lead to issues. If you are cognizant of this fact, you can rest assured that sugar in moderation is *not* evil. So if you have a sweet tooth and feel like maybe trying to live without your daily dose of chocolate is just too overwhelming, then eat your chocolate! Cut or change something else instead.

So, the next question is: how much is "too much" sugar? The American Heart Association recommends that men should consume no more than 9 teaspoons (36 grams or 150 calories) of added sugar per day. For women, the number is lower: 6 teaspoons (25 grams or 100 calories) per day. Take a peek at your labels.. and you are going to see.. that isn't very much at all!!! One container of Dannon Light & Fit nonfat vanilla greek yogurt contains 8 grams of sugar. That is almost ⅓ of the entire daily recommended allowance. And speaking of which... **label reading** is *super duper* important if you are eating foods from a container!!!

I do NOT recommend using artificial sweeteners in place of sugar for sweetening foods. Artificial sweeteners are chemicals made in a lab, and do not belong inside your body! If you really can't do without the sweetening, I recommend raw sugar, brown sugar, raw honey or *real* maple syrup... white sugar if you absolutely *have* to. Avoid high fructose corn syrup, aspartame, saccharin (if that still exists in food these days!) and sucralose, if at all possible. You will need to read labels carefully.. these ingredients hide in MANY foods! As a fan of protein powder and shakes, I even have a hard time finding any without sucralose! Grrrr!

Fasting

This is another one that drives me insane.. the new fasting fad. Let's take a population of undernourished women and advise that they eat even *less*. Fasting is most definitely NOT a "one size fits all" plan. Is it useful in certain cases? I'm sure it is... and I don't disagree with the fact that some of us civilized humans could probably afford to go for periods of time without putting calories in our bodies. But the biggest problem I see with fasting is that most people are not nourishing themselves properly to begin with. If you are eating a balanced and healthy, mostly whole foods diet already, you are healthy and all your "systems" are functioning optimally, and you are *strategically* using fasting to maintain weight or to "mix things up," then, in my opinion, this is an appropriate use of fasting.

If you are already NOT eating properly, have bodily imbalances due to lack of nourishment and decide to "fast" to lose weight.. then absolutely not. You should work towards improving your diet and your health before you turn to eating even less. Fasting is for health-conscious, healthy individuals who know what they are doing and why. It is not a "weight loss plan." You can actually damage your metabolism through the improper use of fasting if you don't know what you are doing.

Alcohol

Alcohol use and abuse is widespread in our social structure... Being a mom, I have become painfully aware of how many songs on the radio refer to alcohol use and abuse. I truly wish it wasn't so glorified.. but also at the same time condemned. The messages we send our children are mixed and confusing. The message seems to be "it's OK to drink and to drink a lot, but not to actually GET DRUNK." Hmmm.. that seems.. difficult? Impossible? I've seen shows geared towards teenagers where the kids are drinking at a party, but yet none of them actually ever get *drunk*. Ok....

I certainly have no advice here as I still haven't figured out how to navigate this one myself. So this is when I say again.. moderation. Alcohol and I have had a love/hate relationship since I was too young to feel comfortable admitting, and as the intensity of hangovers increases by the year, that relationship becomes more and more tenuous. I think quite frequently about giving up alcohol altogether, but whether I like it or not, alcohol does actually bring me joy. I tend to be a "reserved" person by nature, one who does not open up and show herself easily to others and who has antisocial tendencies. Alcohol is one avenue to relaxing, to opening up and being able to connect to others in ways that I cannot otherwise do. Without alcohol, I would have a hard time connecting to others on a social level and it is not my wish to spend more time alone. It allows me to be silly, to talk when I'm usually on the quiet side and maybe even to address issues and talk about things that I may be too shy to talk about otherwise. I have a few good friends that I really enjoy having drinks with because it is an enjoyable experience, and my husband is one of them. Drinking is actually a really fun experience for me; the only issues I have with it are the hangovers/feeling it the next day and that part of me deems my alcohol use as "bad," and so continuing to imbibe causes some internal dialogue that I have not figured out a way to circumvent. I have done some psychological work in this area and I am by no means where I want to be in this area of my life, but at this point, I admit to myself that I like to drink and do it at purposeful times, times where I am having fun and enjoying the company of others. I try to avoid drinking for the purpose of making uncomfortable situations more comfortable or for an emotional outlet, as I found this is a bad tactic and does not work in my favor. I try my best to "moderate," but this is definitely one area in my personal life where I struggle. Big time. I tend to go overboard and binge drink. But I try my best and that is all I can do. Beating myself up only leads to more anxiety. Accepting myself leads to a much happier existence. I prefer the latter and so I am working towards that every day... (At the time of publishing this book, I actually decided to hop off the roller coaster and quit drinking altogether.)

But enough about my own relationship with alcohol.. my thoughts on it are: if you can be disciplined and limit yourself to the recommended one drink/day, then lucky you. Go for it. You can easily clear that in a day. There is some evidence that consumption of MODERATE amounts of alcohol has health benefits, but most people go over and beyond what is considered "moderate." Like medications and herbal therapies, it's one of those things that is *absolutely* dose dependent. There's a VERY fine line between drinking being beneficial and drinking being damaging. Moderate drinking is most accurately defined as: up to 1 drink per day for women and 2 drinks per day for men. A "drink" is further defined as 12 ounces of beer (not a typical pint, which is 16 ounces), 5 ounces of wine (not a giant goblet) or 1.5 ounces of hard liquor (a shot glass and a half). Obviously, some people can handle more or less depending on body type, pre-existing conditions, overall health.. but still. The problem with alcohol, as many of us know, is that it affects inhibition. That makes it hard to stop drinking it once you get started. That means that we are actually not helping our bodies at all, but doing damage instead. If you can't drink "moderately" and have no desire to cut back or stop (my first recommendation, of course!), then just be mindful of the fact that you are likely negatively affecting some of your organs (see diagram). You should seriously consider utilizing ways to give your liver, heart, digestive organs and immune system a boost. Overuse of alcohol also often leads to depression, anxiety and sleep issues, which many women struggle with so... if this is you, you can make it better! Refer to diet section (#1!!!), exercise and supplementing therapies, like properly prescribed herbal therapies, acupuncture, stress management. If you want to quit completely, there is a lot of help out there!

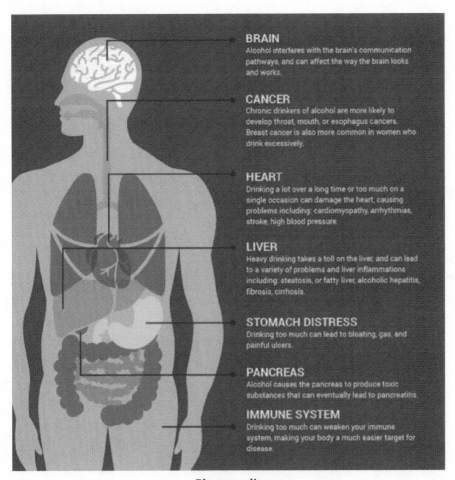

Photo credit:
https://americanaddictioncenters.org/alcoholism-treatment/body-effects

If you are looking to reduce body fat, again, I would recommend quitting or cutting back first, but if that's not in the cards right now, I would stick to drinks that don't contain soda or juices due to the sugar content, and also to drier wines. The sweeter the drink, the more calories it is going to contain for you to have to burn off. And I strongly advise AGAINST drinks with artificial sweeteners like aspartame and sucralose, as is what is contained in "diet," "light" and "sugar-free" drinks. This goes for ANY drink, alcoholic or not. Artificial sweeteners have been linked with all kinds of nasty side effects. Heavy beers should be limited also. Keep in mind that the body tends to use alcohol calories first - they provide more bang for the buck, energy-wise, and they are easier to digest. Add mixers, sugar and heavy hops/wheat and your body will just be burning liquid fuel... forget about any food or excess body fat that you want to get rid of! It can take 1-2 hours just to metabolize one drink, depending on calorie content, size and what kind it is.. more than that and you are looking at several hours. So, in a nutshell, alcohol does not make for a good weight loss plan, to improve health or mood.. but it is a difficult one to contend with due to societal pressures and lack of other effective coping strategies.

Drug & Medications.

Now I realize that this isn't really "diet" per se, but it still qualifies as something external that you are putting in your body. And it's actually a VERY important topic. This topic is a bit taboo for me in my own private practice. This is because as a licensed medical professional in the State of New York, prescribing and advising on pharmaceuticals are not with my "scope of practice." "So I have to advise any patient needing advice on pharmaceuticals to seek advice from their physician" is my usual (and unfortunate) statement when it comes to that. Luckily, you are not seeking my advice in a patient/practitioner relationship, so I will freely share my opinions on this topic. We are a highly OVER-medicated culture. Over the counter and prescription drugs are **destroying** people's bodies, and I believe this with every fiber of my being. Treating patients over the last 10 years has only solidified my stance on this. The potent chemicals that are contained within drugs have no place in our bodies, and chronic use of them is extremely damaging. This even applies to OTC meds like ibuprofen (Advil) and acetaminophen (Tylenol)! Just because you can buy them in the store does not mean they are not toxic. I have seen patients struggle for months to recover from damage done by one medication. Not all patients' bodies are tolerant of such strong chemicals. Imagine taking multiple medications. I can give you a list of reasons why most of the medications taken regularly by patients are actually damaging their bodies. Sure, they may be managing their symptoms, but they are causing other problems. More severe problems. I wholly disagree with modern medicine's method of medicating and I believe that this is contributing to the decline of overall health in this country. Drugs do not FIX issues within the body. They simply treat symptoms. If you don't figure out **why** you are having symptoms and actually solve *that* problem, then you have no hope of ever being symptom-free and you will always have to rely on medications to feel better. So you have high blood pressure. WHY do you have high blood pressure? Blood pressure medication simply reduces your blood pressure but does not fix the REASON your blood pressure is high (which is probably lifestyle!). How about acid reflux? Do you know that many meds for GERD are only meant to be taken for a short time? That is because they damage the digestive environment by neutralizing stomach acid (which we NEED to digest our food). This actually worsens the digestive problems. But patients are often not informed of this. Taking a medication to cover up your symptoms while not actually solving the problem is NOT a long term solution. It is a way to make you dependent on pharmaceuticals and it is most likely causing long term damage to your body.

I recommend a **very** conservative use of of drugs, whether your doctor gives it to you or you buy it at the store. If you do use it, use it minimally. Read the inserts. Know what you are taking and **WHY** you are taking it! Be informed. What is the long term plan? There is definitely a time and a place! Ibuprofen should be used a few times a YEAR, NOT a few times a week. In MOST cases, other tools should be used instead. Many issues can be corrected through lifestyle changes and/or through the use of safer therapies, more than most people realize. All other options should be exhausted, in my opinion. There are many other tools to treat a variety of health issues, other than to put chemicals inside of your body. *Your body should be coveted and cared for, and this is the opposite of that. It deserves better.*

Get Comfy With Your Body Type

I wanted to say a bit about this because I too often see women struggling against their genetics. I see it more often in younger women, but it's still an issue that plagues the female population. Because we are individuals and very different in many ways even from each other, we all contain within us differing genetics that control the shape and tendencies of our bodies. A good indication of your genetics is to take a look at the frames of your parents. Children tend to take on the build of one parent or the other. For example, you will see women who are quite thin with smaller frames and less "flesh," you will see women who are larger framed and have a lot of muscle mass (more of athletic build), and you will see women whose bodies are more "curvy", more "fleshy", the type that will feel like they gain weight if they eat even one sugary treat. Most often, you will see women who are a mixture of these 3 "types." It is important to know this information so that you can know what you can change and what you cannot change. It is also yet *another* reason why there is no "one size fits all" life plan. Diet and exercise are always important and they can certainly be used to "be the best you".. but if you are using either (or both) to try to be a body type that you are not, I am sorry to say that no matter what you do, it isn't going to happen. Not without sacrificing your health and wellbeing, at least. You will just cause yourself mental anguish, and no one needs more of that. That is what we are trying to reduce!

These types have scientific "names," actually. They are called ectomorphs, mesomorphs and endomorphs. See the diagram below for visual reference.

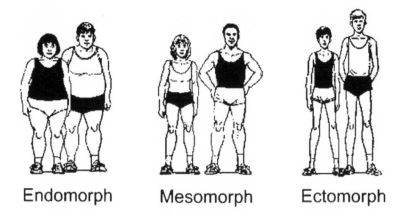

Photo Reference:
https://blog.ekincare.com/2016/05/19/what-body-type-are-you/

Ectomorphs have smaller frames, smaller bone structures, less "flesh" (muscle and fat). They tend to be our *Victoria's Secret* models and our long distance runners. They have fast metabolisms as their bodies do not store fat easily. They also do not build muscle easily. If ectomorphs want to build muscle and strength, they have to try very hard. They have a tendency to *lose* flesh easily: muscle and fat, so athletes of this body type have to always make sure they are taking in enough calories. These are the ones that lose weight "on accident."

Mesomorphs tend to be more "medium-framed" with medium bone structures. They develop muscle mass easily and usually have more muscle than fat on their bodies. They have what many sources call "a rectangular frame," meaning that shoulders, waist and hips tend to be in line with one another; they are not overly "curvy" in the midsection and hips. Mesomorphs have the muscle-building advantage as they do this quite easily, but they can also gain fat just as easily. This means they have to be much more conscientious about diet and exercise if they do not want to gain too much body fat.

Endomorphs have larger body frames, are "bigger boned." They are softer and more "curvy" and tend to carry more body fat than the other types. Think J Lo and Marilyn Monroe! The fat distribution usually centers around the waist, hips and thighs. They are typically smaller in the upper body, while larger in the lower body, making them what many sources refer to as "pear shaped." "From a metabolic perspective, endomorph body types usually have some degree of carbohydrate and insulin sensitivity." (U Rock Girl!, 2014).

And there it is... yet ANOTHER diet complexity! Body types matter too!!! Another reason why "one size fits all" diet plans do not work for everyone. Because ectomorphs have blazing fast metabolisms, they can eat just about anything they want and not gain weight. As I mentioned earlier, ectomorphs that WANT to gain size and muscle mass have to work really hard at it because this group is known as the "hard gainers." This group should NEVER fast!! They should eat plenty of protein, healthy fats and healthy carbohydrates, regardless of source. Since their muscle mass is lower than in the other types, their protein requirements are not as high. On the other hand, mesomorphs have a higher protein requirement because they have muscular builds. Higher protein diets work better for mesomorphs. This group should take their carbohydrate intake down a smidge and focus more on protein and healthy fat. Endomorphs often have a problem metabolizing high-glycemic, starchy carbohydrates so this group should stick to more whole fruit & vegetable carbohydrate sources and limit grain sources (flours, rice, etc). The "Paleo" diet that I mentioned earlier works great for this group. "Lower carb" is definitely a go here.

Most people are a combination of two types, with one being more dominant. I am a meso-endomorph. My type is more dominantly a mesomorph, but I have the endomorphic tendencies towards gaining fat in my middle, hips and thighs. I have an athletic build, I'm strong and I gain muscle easily, but I also gain fat easily. I have muscular arms and legs, which tends to make some clothes fit oddly on me. My body does not lose flesh easily. This is great when it comes to muscle mass. But when it comes to body fat, I have to work very hard and be very diligent with diet in order to lose it, and it takes a looong time. High protein, "paleo" diet works best for me. I most definitely gain weight when I eat too many grain sources of carbohydrates. To be honest, even I sometimes have a hard time embracing my own body type. I really desire to have less body fat and to be leaner, especially in the midsection and rear area. I don't actually feel like I *look* like I work out as much as I do and that I work as hard at eating as healthfully as I do.. Our own body images are distorted and that is part of the problem. It's that "expectations" thing again. You can work and work, but will you ever even realize when you're "there?" I have had people call me "tiny," "jacked" - I have never felt like I was either of those things. I still feel like I am constantly fighting to keep the fat from accumulating.

So that leads me to this question: if you do have a bodily goal, what is it? It is important that any goals you have for your body are realistic. Scale weight is a common goal because it is easy to measure (and we are trained to care about the number), but contrary to how the medical community makes you feel, scale weight is NOT an accurate measurement and it actually shouldn't be used to assess one's body composition. Once upon a time, someone somewhere came up with this ratio of weight to height (called the BMI, or body mass index) that puts you on some arbitrary chart to see where you stack up against "everyone else", I guess. (This is why you get measured and weighed when you go to the doctor. So your BMI can go in your chart.) The problem with this system? How can one extremely simplified number apply to an entire population of individuals? And who decided what is "normal," "healthy," making people who lie outside this range feel like they have to strive to get into it? Ok, so maybe I'm a little bitter... ever since I started purposely building muscle mass in my 20s, I have fallen into the "overweight" category on the BMI chart. My weight oscillates between 140 and 150lbs and I am just over 5'2." So when I think about it, "overweight" is really a simple term. It simply means that something weighs more than some predetermined number. It's just a word and shouldn't be associated with anything good or bad... but it is. "Overweight" is a less than desirable thing to be in the medical community. In fact, the definition of "overweight" when it comes to the Mayo Clinic is "Weight above what's considered healthy, often measured using body mass index (BMI)." Hmmmmmm.

Here's a little history lesson on that BMI number. It was originally created in the 1830s. 1830s!! Almost 200 years ago! It was created for the purpose of measuring *populations* for the assessment of public health and comparison to other populations, NOT for the individuals. Yet, this number is still widely used across the American medical community. In fact, if your number falls into the "obese" BMI range, you will now be labeled with the diagnosis of "obesity". In 1998, the BMI values were updated - lowered, actually... putting over 50% of the population into the overweight or obese category! "A particular problem with BMI as an index of obesity is that it does not differentiate between body lean mass and body fat mass; that is, a person can have a high BMI but still have a very low fat mass and vice versa." (Nutall, 2015) Like me! So, it is a wonder why we all feel like we need to "lose weight"? I'm an athlete with a great diet and I'm still "overweight"!!

So forget the damn scale. Body fat reduction is a bit better goal, but harder to accurately measure. If you have a scale with the ability to measure body fat, you can use that *as a visual guide* to gauge progress if you are actively trying to "lose". Few readily available body fat measurement tools are overly accurate. You can hop on for the first time, measure it and then take it from there. Is your goal a certain pants' size? Given that women's pants sizes are different across different manufacturers, this is like aiming for a moving target. Try not to get too emotionally attached to numbers, good or bad. Numbers are just numbers. YOU are the one that attaches feelings and emotions to them, but you can change that. You can change your expectations, just like I wrote about earlier.

Maybe instead of aiming for a specific number, you go by how you *feel* in your own skin. "My goal is to be comfortable in my own skin." For me, my range is intuitive. I start getting a little lax on my diet and I start feeling a bit more puffy, my clothes start fitting a little tighter and I start grabbing my upper size limit clothes off the shelf. I *know* that I have been slacking and that I can do better, and I feel not so confident in my own skin. I get tired of that after awhile, so I rein in my eating and get down to work. About 5 lbs less and I am comfortable again, and in the smaller sizes. I have been doing this for a long time, so I know. I recognize that there is a point where I feel content, and there is a point where I don't. And it has nothing to do with any numbers. Also, don't forget that old saying "muscle weighs more than fat." It's true. And muscle is denser and more compact, so more muscular people are naturally going to weigh more. I'm not saying it's not super fun to watch numbers go down when you are working hard. It's validating. Just try not to take it seriously and let it disrupt your inner peace. It isn't worth that.

Don't let someone else's attachment to arbitrary numbers dictate where YOU feel comfortable. I STILL fight off the "150lbs is too heavy for my size" and then I have to remind myself that it ISN'T. It must not be. I do all the right things. I weigh what I weigh. My weight is just a meaningless number, and *someone else* decided whether it was "too high," "too low," or "just right." Damn you, Goldilocks!! The important thing is that I feel confident and healthy, and that is what's most important.

Guess What? We Menstruate!

A h.. and at last, the "real" reason why men's health and wellness recommendations do not apply to women... because we bleed every month and birth children. Our physiology is NOT THE SAME as a man's physiology, and therefore, our dietary needs are different. It frustrates me that in this day and age, and all the focus on "equality" that there is still so little widespread information on the nutritional needs of women due to their unique physiology. A WOMAN'S PHYSIOLOGY IS TOTALLY DIFFERENT THAN A MAN'S. Do I need to say that again? In the words of Stacy Sims: "Women are not small men." (If you are an athlete and you haven't read her book "ROAR," then you really need to!!!)

Obviously it goes without saying that our menstrual cycles are a HUGE part of our lives as women. Depending on how you were raised, you may even have some cultural or religious beliefs, certain emotions (likely negative) or even *shame* attached to menstruating. Menstruation is a completely normal and healthy function of the female human body, and it should be viewed that way! And it's a big deal in a woman's life, not something that should be swept under the rug.

Our internal physiology changes and cycles every single *month* and yet, many women are so detached and unaware of what is actually happening within their own bodies. Therefore, I think it's important to give an overview so that we can fully understand what is happening and how it relates to how WE feel and in turn, to what actions we take on a daily basis.

In Chinese medicine, the menstrual cycle is divided into 4 different parts. Using a 28 day cycle as a broad example since many women's menstrual cycles are about that long, each 7 day block represents a different time in the cycle in which different processes are occurring. (Also note that *cycle length* is defined as the first day of menses until the last day before the next menses).

The "blood" phase: This phase is the time when women are physically bleeding. During this time, the hormone levels (specifically estrogen and progesterone) are at their lowest. Most importantly, women are losing actual blood right now, so blood that used to be available inside the body is now leaving the body. So, think about this for a second: we lose a decent volume of blood EVERY month. So EVERY month, we need to recoup this blood we are using (or eventually we would just run dry, right? No joke, though - this is ACTUALLY the cause of many health issues in older women!) In addition, some organ systems (such as the liver and uterus) are working harder than usual. Women may feel fatigued, crampy, nauseous, bloated, experience headaches or some combination of these during this time. Technically, this is the time of month when women should actually take it *easy*, especially if they tend towards having what we Chinese medicine practitioners call a "blood or yin (fluid) deficiency." During this time, women should definitely NOT be fasting, should be eating a diet rich in "blood building" foods and should be trying their best to take it easier than normal, at least traditionally... but we're Americans! We scoff at rest, and life doesn't stop for a woman's menstrual cycle! Therein lies part of the chronicity of women's health problems. And this is all because we need to rebuild that blood I mentioned earlier... and most often, we don't! Women vary highly in their experiences during menses. Some bleed more heavily, more lightly, for longer or shorter periods (no pun intended!). Some have painful periods and other breeze right through. Typically, menses should last about 5-7 days, with it getting naturally shorter as the woman gets older. Periods that are too heavy or too light, or are too short or too long indicate that a woman's system is out of balance. Most women don't complain about periods that are too light or too short... until they want to get pregnant, and then this is a real problem. Periods that are too light or too short may mean that she is not building an adequate uterine lining, and this is IMPERATIVE for a successful pregnancy. If women are losing too much blood every month, this is a serious problem, as month after month of this will eventually take its toll and reflect in her overall health. I would consider "too much" bleeding if a woman is bleeding for more than 7 days in a month consistently.

The "yin" phase: "Yin" in Chinese medicine is loosely translated as "fluid", meaning the wet, watery substance required by the body for various functions. This phase is the time between when the woman ceases bleeding and when ovulation occurs. Ovulation typically occurs around 14 days *before* menses. So, for a 28 day cycle, ovulation "typically" occurs around day 14. Obviously, this varies between women. If they pay attention, many women will notice signs of ovulation, such as cramping, cervical mucus/discharge that looks like egg white. There may be an increase in libido leading up to it (that's the body's way of trying to foster procreation!). During this time, estrogen levels are high and progesterone levels are low. The body is busily trying to make and accumulate rich, nutrient-filled blood to send to the uterus to make the endometrial lining for possible implantation of a fertilized egg. Once ovulation occurs, production of the uterine lining ceases, so this is THE week when that lining is built. Maybe, if you are not actively trying to get pregnant, you don't really care about the quality of the uterine lining.. but if you DO want to get pregnant, either now or in the future, caring about the quality of this lining is something you are going to want to do.

The "yang" phase: "Yang" in Chinese medicine relates more to the non-tangible activities. In this case, it refers to the "warming" that occurs as a results of increased progesterone production. This phase occurs between ovulation and about a week before menses. An egg is released from an ovary at ovulation and the egg will begin to travel through the fallopian tube and into the uterus. Progesterone levels rise and women physically become almost a full degree warmer then they are during the first two phases. This is because embryos need it warmer to continue growth and development. Women who tend to be more heat sensitive may notice an increase in hot flashes, night sweating, disruption in sleep and energy levels, maybe irritability and just generally feel different than usual. Women who are more sensitive to cold may actually be more comfortable during this time. While yang is actually many things, one thing that yang is, is heat. If you are a woman that tends to run cold, you may notice that during this phase of your cycle, you may be less sensitive to cold. A decrease in libido will likely begin during this time and last up until the beginning of menses. This is normal. Think about it.. sex is craved because the woman's body needs sperm to fertilize an egg, and this process only occurs pre-ovulation. By the time ovulation occurs, this biological need ceases. In fact, the body undergoes changes to "lock down" entrance to the uterus in order to protect a fertilized embryo, and even changes the pH of the uterus to kill off any potential invaders and tightens up the cervical opening. It's really quite a slick system! So if you are feeling less sexual desire during the second half of your menstrual cycle, you can be assured (and assure your partner, which I have to do repeatedly, I can assure YOU!) that is the way nature intended it!

The "qi" (pronounced "chee") phase: The word "qi" in this case refers to the egg moving from the ovary to the uterus and to the chemical reactions and responses that occur which determine if the egg has been fertilized and will implant into the uterine lining. A lot of really important stuff is happening here! About a week after ovulation and assuming that pregnancy didn't occur, the woman's body will know that fertilization did not occur and now it has to release the egg and the endometrial lining that it has saved up and essentially "reset" back to square one. If the woman is, in fact, pregnant, the body will initiate a whole other set of chemical processes. This is essentially a decision tree, and the actions the body takes depends on the presence or absence of hormonal signals. In Chinese medicine theory, the liver is responsible for a majority of the work that is done here and this is the time that a lot of women suffer from PMS symptoms: food cravings, emotional changes, bloating, headaches, breast tenderness, cramping, sleep issues, night sweats.... The body is actually doing a lot of work internally and it may leave you feeling fatigued, irritable, feeling down and/or in pain, especially if your liver is already struggling to keep up with the demands of "normal" life. Imagine if you are just barely coping with the duties of day-to-day life and then suddenly, your boss throws a big project at you. At this time, you'll have to prioritize and likely, some area of your life will get neglected (maybe even this "project") while you cope with the new demands on you. This is exactly what your liver feels like during this phase of your menstrual cycle. Unfortunately for most of us, due to the constant barrage of both internal and external toxins, our livers are just barely squeaking by on a normal day. This is why PMS is such a common syndrome for many women. But PMS isn't really "normal," or healthy, especially if it is interfering with aspects of your life. It can and should be resolved.

Women's menstrual health is an extremely good indicator of women's general health. The menstrual cycle is a VERY normal and VERY needed process when it comes to women's physiology. Menstrual blood release is a woman's way of expelling toxins and keeping her normal, cyclical physiology flowing normally. When women don't bleed, bleed irregularly or too heavily, this is a problem that needs to be addressed. Unfortunately, the way this is typically addressed by Western medicine practitioners is to use birth control to regulate the woman's hormones and therefore, her menstruation. The biggest issue with this is that the birth control actually takes over the woman's cycle artificially and DOES NOT CORRECT the problems that caused irregularities in the first place. In many cases, certain forms of birth control even stop a woman from bleeding altogether. This is a problem because the release of blood during menses is one of the ways a woman's body releases "toxins." Believe it or not, it is also a "cleansing" process! Often, when women decide to come off birth control (usually to achieve pregnancy), the same issues will return. In addition, long term use of birth control can be detrimental to a woman's health. Some studies have shown a link between oral birth control and breast cancer (Kumle, M, et al., 2002), and also that the longer a woman is on them, the higher the risk becomes.

Keep in mind that even as humans, we are STILL animals on earth and the #1 biological priority of every living thing on this planet is procreation. Therefore, every physiological system contained in every organism is wired for procreation and proliferation, first and foremost. Just because we've gotten separated from our "wild" side doesn't make us any different. So what does that mean? That means that the #1 priority of women's bodies is to achieve and maintain pregnancy. This will still occur even when a woman has internal deficiencies. Hormonal changes, coupled with dietary deficiencies, can cause a woman's body to actually FEED off of itself to maintain the reproductive system and the same holds true during pregnancy. The fetus will almost always get what it needs, but it's the women's body that will suffer if she is not taking care to get what she needs to maintain herself (and a fetus if she is pregnant). This is totally different from men, whose bodies have no reason to do that. Men are not the givers of life. And therefore, their needs are far different than ours.

So if I have menstrual problems, how do I deal with them? You ask. Well, hopefully this book will help some. Then I recommend seeking out a practitioner trained in more holistic approaches to the body: Chinese medicine, ayurveda, functional medicine. You need to find a practitioner who can help you by using medication as a last option. Lifestyle changes are very important: diet, exercise, and stress management can go a long way. Herbal supplementation can also be very helpful but you need to be guided by a trained professional. There is too much self-prescribing when it comes to herbs and supplements and this is not a good thing. Just because one supplement worked for your friend doesn't mean that it is appropriate and will work for you. Humans are too different from one another for any cure to be a "one size fits all."

And Then We Stop (Menopause)

Shouldn't it be called "menostop??"

Contrary to cultural opinion, menopause is actually a GOOD thing. The woman's body gets to stop the cycling, the blood dumping and rebuilding every month, which means... she gets to FINALLY build and retain the blood nourishment that the body's tissues desperately need. In ancient Chinese culture and medicine, menopausal women are the wise ones, the "sages." This is because, instead of blood leaving the body every single month, the blood gets to stay in the body and continue to build to nourish the brain (and everywhere else!). It is NOT the end of life. It is the beginning of a whole new chapter, just like childhood up until puberty. A new phase.

Culturally, we view menopause as a negative thing. "All dried up". It should, in fact, be the opposite. It's a time to rest and rebuild. Most women reach menopause around their mid-50s. The *average* life expectancy of a woman in the US today is 78 years old. So most of us have another 25+ years of life left AFTER we reach menopause... and we don't have to be subject to our menstrual ups and downs, and bleed anymore. It should be a celebration, in my opinion.

Menopause, for many women, can bring a lot of discomfort with it (physical and emotional). It is very similar to the issues that surround the menstrual cycle that I mentioned earlier. Women who experience hormonal imbalances and discomfort around their menses are much more likely to suffer from menopausal discomfort, if they don't get their issues under control earlier in life. Just like with menses, menopause is *not* SUPPOSED to be a time filled with unbearable hot flashes, insomnia, irritability and anxiety. If it is, you can can and SHOULD seek help. You have some hormonal imbalances that can be straightened out and then you will be a lot happier. I recommend working holistically to deal with them through the lifestyle changes and not through hormone replacement. Just like with birth control pills, hormone replacement does not **fix** issues and it *does* increase your chances of getting cancer.

This is DEFINITELY the time to take better care of your physical, mental and emotional self. So take the time and do it, because it's now or never!

Go With The Flow

As women, we are essentially biologically driven by our menstrual cycles. Most women don't even know that. Hormones control not only the way we feel physically, but they can control our emotions and our moods, which in turn drives our actions.

For example, now that I am in my mid-40s, I can say this about me during my cycle: The first half of my cycle is my favorite time. I am positive, ideas are flowing, my mind is clearer. I am in love with my husband, am not easily annoyed by him and am definitely more apt to desire sex during this time. I have energy. I sleep well. Life is good and I am not worrying about how everything good could just crash and burn in an instant. I feel strong and lean and more confident in my own skin. I once joked that I needed to schedule my new patient appointments and speaking engagements around my menstrual cycle. I definitely have an easier time finding words, and my mind is less likely to go blank during the first half of my menstrual cycle. I often wish I could perpetually stay in that phase. Life is so much more pleasant during that time. I am hopeful that this is what menopause will be like!!!

Once ovulation comes, things start to go south in a hurry. I start finding myself getting annoyed more quickly by my husband and even my beloved dogs, and I just want to be left alone (although I don't ever verbalize this). I get snappy and frustrated merely by conversation. I start to worry more. About everything. My workouts feel hard and I feel weaker and discouraged. I feel more bloated, softer and my clothes get tighter and that makes me MORE discouraged. I get logy, tired, less productive and even my brain function is less sharp than it can be.

Approximately one week before my menses, I have started to notice that I feel like a caged animal in my own life, bound by the constructs of my "supposed-tos," "have-tos" and even "want-tos," to a certain degree. I hate my usual life routine and the mundane tasks that accompany it. All I want to do is run away. I literally fantasize about moving to another country and will seal the deal on vacations during these days. I probably even signed up for my Ironman in Mexico during one of these weeks! My husband's small talk about work infuriates me. Cooking dinner infuriates me. Even the need to eat infuriates me! I don't want to clean the house, do laundry, even be at home. I want to be free. I find it interesting that in Muslim culture, women are to avoid men during menstruation and keep to themselves. Some opinions are that this is a "punishment." Does this sound like a "punishment"?

The extremely interesting part of this.. at least to me... is that in Chinese medicine theory, the liver organ "does not like to be constrained," which means that the liver needs to move and flow freely in order to do its job.. and the liver is HIGHLY active during this part of the menstrual cycle. So the fact that, for whatever reason, I feel more resistant to being "constrained" myself during this time, is absolutely appropriate when it comes to Chinese medicine theory. Apparently my liver wants to be "free" during this time. I don't actually know what that translates into from a life perspective. I haven't gotten that part figured out yet. I do know that its intensity changes seasonally, likely due to extra constraints placed on my life by the climate, my daughter's school schedule and my husband's diminished vacation time. November and December seem to be the worst. More social "rules" and "supposed-tos" during this time than any other during the year. What to do about it all this is a different story. I honestly haven't figured out a good way to combat it, short of abandoning my life for a week a month. Alcohol helps to alleviate the discomfort, but isn't really a healthy option in my opinion. I historically drink WAY TOO MUCH during the holidays, in an attempt to not be a miserable person. Holidays are stressful and NOT joyful for many women! No, it's not the best coping mechanism and I would never advise a patient to use it. But I'm human, like everyone else, and still continue to improve my own life coping mechanisms.

I have found that getting outside definitely helps. During these times I usually dream of the beach or hiking in the woods. Obviously that is a much healthier option, but unfortunately can be a bit less accessible depending on life scheduling and weather. Living in upstate New York, it's a bit of a challenge to just zip off to a warm beach when my daughter is in school all week long, and on top of that, being a divorced parent brings a whole new level of complexity to spontaneous travel.

Most women don't keep track of their cycles like I do, but I find that I am less likely to experience anxiety surrounding my symptoms when I know that I can attribute my less desirable bodily and mood changes to hormonal fluctuations during my menstrual cycle. I recommend keeping track, maybe jotting notes down in a journal, so that women can see what happens to them physically, emotionally and mentally throughout the cycle. I often ask my patients, "Where are you in your menstrual cycle?" It matters!!! A pattern will become more obvious to you as time goes by, and know that what you're feeling and doing is probably biologically appropriate. It is important to be as introspective as you can, but it's complicated so it takes time and consistency. YOU are complicated. We all are. Forgive yourself if you are feeling tired or cranky, and know that "this, too, shall pass." Also know that if you are actually suffering as a result of your menstrual cycle, you CAN make changes that will help you. Refer back to the section on diet first and foremost. Then proceed from there.

Even though we are supposed to be in modern times, we are STILL caught up in old ideas, ideas that men have formed about women, their bodies and their minds! Oftentimes, I recognize the fact that we are nowhere near as "modern" as we seem to think we are. It is STILL not socially acceptable for women to have "mood swings." Changes in mood are a NORMAL part of a woman's physiology!! See the next section! We are creatures that change about every week of every month. But yet, aren't many of us taught, directly or indirectly, that is not acceptable to act in any other way other than to be agreeable, "rational", selfless... certainly not "moody," "bitchy," "hormonal," "irrational," "frigid" (do they still use that word??), "bossy." For Gods' sake, my ex-husband still thinks women should be selfless and not have needs of their own.. which is why he is my "ex" husband now. I can't count how many times he's called me "selfish" throughout the years; "selfish" for pursuing my dreams and for treating myself like a person worthy of being taken care of.

As women, I feel that we are expected **not** to change mentally and emotionally, despite the fact that we undergo physiological hormonal changes approximately every 7 days, that we are "supposed to" function like we are not changing at all. That we are like men (who do also undergo hormonal changes, but the effects tend to be more subtle than in women.) As a result, we get stressed when we change and so do those around us. We think there is something wrong with us. So we find coping mechanisms to help tame that dragon in us that sometimes wants to come out, but we are too afraid to let it... because it isn't "socially acceptable," and we don't want to take it out on our families. Alcohol? Eating? Or not eating? Prescription drugs? Smoking? Over-exercise? Is this maybe the reason that women and wine seem to be synonyms for so many women I know? Many women are raised to think they don't even deserve to take the time or money to care for themselves! All of this is still so common that it infuriates me. "Modern," huh?

Hormones Affect Emotions. (No, We're Not Crazy!)

When researching for this book, I was really taken aback (although not surprised) about how *little* research has been done regarding the relationship between emotions and fluctuations in sex hormones. In fact, one 2018 psychology journal explicitly states, "To date, no research has investigated whether sex hormones are associated with emotion regulation in women." (Graham, et al., 2018). NO RESEARCH?! I've researched a zillion things in my life and very seldom have come up empty-handed, but to come up empty-handed on a topic as huge and as important as this? Given the fact that the incidence of anxiety and depression is 2-3x higher in women for some "unknown reason?" I'm officially speechless. This is the point at which I realize that we need more women in the research and medical fields....

Luckily, we don't rely much on research when it comes to living our daily lives. As women, we know darn well from our menstruating experiences that our emotional and mental states *do* change in response to our menstrual cycles. As I mentioned earlier, keep a journal. Validate the fact that your emotions do *indeed* change through your cycle and get in touch with the more "animal" side of yourself, because that is in fact what you are.

If you think for a second about the purpose of the menstrual cycle, we can simplify it into the following actions: 1- create a nourishing lining in the uterus for a fertilized egg to implant into and begin its development, 2- create a fertile environment to welcome sperm and keep the environment hospital to them, 3- release an egg and help egg and sperm meet for fertilization, 4- when fertilization occurs, protect the fertilized egg by shifting the environment so as to make it more comfortable for the fertilized egg and less so for any potential threat to the egg (other sperm, viruses, bacteria, external objects), 5- implant and shut down so that the embryo can grow and develop.

This seems obvious and simple, right? Now think about how the chemicals involved in this process might shift your emotions to assist in procreation. Assuming you are a fairly healthy woman with a fairly normal menstrual cycle, you are going to be a lot more open and relaxed physically, mentally and emotionally before ovulation occurs. You need connection, sex, sperm.

That is what the body is seeking. Then ovulation occurs and everything begins to shift over the next few days. From a reproductive standpoint, your body has everything it needs to complete the rest of the cycle (with the exception of food) - you may actually find that you are hungrier during the second half of your cycle and this is when the food cravings may begin to set in. As I mentioned earlier, you may shut down a bit physically, mentally and emotionally. Reducing stimulation allows the body to put more energy into the second half of the cycle. Doesn't this make perfect sense?

There are actual physiological REASONS for the emotional changes that occur over the course of your monthly menstrual cycle and sometimes these emotional changes are unpleasant and may not mesh well into your normal daily activities. Maybe your premenstrual week lies right over Thanksgiving, and instead of feeling joyful about the holiday, you are feeling anxious and irritable, you want to run away and you are frustrated that you decided to prepare dinner for a whole group of people... Does this mean that your emotions are pathological, that you are "wrong" to feel irritable when you "should" be happy about the holiday? Absolutely not! And how many times have women gotten down on themselves for feeling a different way than they think the situation warrants? And then what? Too much wine? Medication? A panic attack? A total meltdown in the kitchen, or snapping at family members? It isn't our emotions themselves that cause us problems, it's the fact that we get to be grown ass women with packed lives before we even realize that we have no idea how to cope with these kinds of situations. That nobody told most of us that it is OK to be "emotional," so instead of accepting it and acknowledging it and being OK with it, we try to ignore it; we shove our feelings inside, and smile instead of screaming at someone like we really want to. THIS IS NOT OK. AND IT IS NOT HEALTHY. It leads to unhealthy coping strategies, like addiction and mental health issues. Some might also argue, especially those of us in the practice of holistic health, that continuously holding in your emotions leads to chronic physical conditions, like cancer, stroke and cardiovascular disease. In fact, there is QUITE a bit of research on this topic. Many studies show a link between chronic emotion suppression and mortality. One such study was conducted by joint efforts of the University of Rochester Medical Center and the Harvard School of Public Health, and the findings were as follows:

"Our analysis of a US nationally representative sample, followed for 12 years for mortality by cause of death, revealed significant associations between higher levels of emotion suppression and all-cause as well as cancer-related mortality. These findings have several implications. Theoretically, suppression is presumed to promote unhealthy behaviors as a substitute for appropriate emotional expression, and possibly engender neuroendocrine dysregulation" (Chapman, et al., 2013).

So, great point, right? If you are good at suppressing your emotions, you are probably engaging in less than healthy behaviors in order to be successful at it. So, fine. It's probably fair to say that many of us are doing that. But if you are aware of it and it is something that you are interested in improving, there are certainly avenues for that. I'm hoping that is why you are reading this book! So we can help to balance the bad with the good! And maybe do a better job coping, so as to use less of the "bad," right? Right!

My advice to you is to get in touch with, and I mean REALLY in touch, with your menstrual cycle and the physical, mental and emotional changes that take place during it. So again... journal! It will take time, but it will help. It is very possible that not every month will be the same. The weather, the season, your current life situation... these things are going to affect your menstrual cycle. Yes, external factors DO affect our own internal bodily processes. Maybe you are more irritable in the winter because you can't get out as much and the days are shorter.. or maybe you have more insomnia in the summer because of the heat. Sometimes even our cycles lengthen or shorten on different intervals or seasons. Everyone is a bit different.

The Importance of Exercise

I believe that if there is ONE thing you do for yourself and for your health, it is to eat healthfully. Choose wisely. Give yourself the permission to treat yourself as if you are important, because guess what?? YOU ARE. I have no doubt that you have amazing things to contribute to this world and that you make a lasting impact on the lives of others, be it friends, family, co-workers, clients/patients, maybe even complete strangers. I am sure some of them would agree that you are worth putting the energy into taking care of!

The next best thing you can do for your body is to make sure it gets to move the way it was designed to move. If you don't, it will stop moving and it will start hurting, and you will not like it. It's that simple.

Have you ever heard the term "move it or lose it?" This saying is never more appropriate than it is for the human body. I've said this before, but our bodies are amazing. They are so incredibly adaptable. Most people in the modern world have no idea to what extent our bodies can endure and adapt, as we are able to avoid harsh conditions and don't have to go too far or too long without food. We're quite spoiled, to be fair. But I'm sure you've seen stories about people who have survived some pretty crazy situations or about people who have completed athletic feats that most people cannot possibly fathom. Completing a full Ironman was a big one for me. I could not possibly imagine that my body could swim 2.4 miles, ride 112 miles on a bike and then run 26.2 miles.. all in one day... but it happened because I spent time conditioning my body, purposely causing *adaptation* so I could complete it. Athletes do this all the time. It is the whole basis for their training; the REASON they go to practice. They are intentionally forcing their bodies to adapt, and they do and will.

The opposite is true for people who don't exercise at all. Muscle and bone mass will decrease, and so will the blood flow to them; these are "expensive" tissues for the body to maintain and so the body will let go of what is not being used, and just keep around the bare minimum. It's like having a fancy car in the garage that you don't drive. Why pay insurance, fees and maintenance on something that you barely drive? Our bodies can function through an average person's daily routine with a minimal amount of effort, and it gets more and more efficient each day that it does the same routine. It adapts. It actually *changes* itself, its structure, to be able to use the minimal amount of resources and effort that it possibly can to complete a task or a series of tasks. This is why you may have heard, when it comes to exercise, that you should always be changing up what you are doing.. so that the body does not have a chance to adapt.

I think what most people don't realize is that the body is SUPER dynamic; it is *always* growing, changing, dying, regenerating.. every second of every day. Some parts grow and change faster than others. Think about the turnover for your hair and nails, for example. And even this changes based on your lifestyle. The more repetitive it is, the larger the degree of adaptation.

Now, if your body is only conditioned to move in certain ways, when it is asked to move in ways it isn't used to, it is going to complain, most likely in the form of pain. This is often where injuries come in. Think for a minute about the motion involved in your legs during walking, most notably the upper legs and thighs. Mostly, they go forward and backward during walking, motions that we in the medical field call flexion and extension, respectively. Now your upper leg actually moves in 6 different directions. Other than forward and backwards (flexion and extension), it also moves side to side, called adduction (towards your midline) and abduction (away from your midline), and it also rotates outwards and inwards (called external rotation and internal rotation). So say for "exercise," you mostly just walk or stand, whether purposely for exercise or just life activities, and your legs aren't used to moving in a side-to-side or rotational manner (because you don't engage in activities that require that). One day, during a fine winter day, you slip in an icy parking lot and your leg suddenly slips out to the side. Soon after, you have pain and begin limping. You now have a muscle strain to deal with that may last for weeks. Maybe you have a tendon tear that occurred because your muscles were not equipped to deal with the sudden new motion that the slip elicited. My point is that maybe you feel like you are able to easily accomplish your usual activities, but don't forget.. things happen suddenly that we have no control over, and it is important to keep your body as strong and flexible as it can possibly be so you don't end up having to make a hospital visit for a slip.. or even a sneeze! It is not only inconvenient, it can be costly, especially when you get surgeries involved. I have seen many, *many* patients who experience years of pain from one simple incident. Maybe they picked up a box the wrong way or they slipped and fell on a wet floor. I am not saying you can prevent everything, but strong and flexible bodies can withstand a lot more.

One of my patients asked me once why I thought older adults tend to suffer from more injuries in their rotator cuff muscles (the muscles around the shoulder). It happens from disuse. When our shoulders are not moved in all the ways they are designed to move, not only does the muscle mass and circulation around them decrease, but the scapula will *actually* start to adhere to the rib cage. This is what is known as "frozen shoulder," and actually results in the shoulder not being ABLE to move. Try to move a shoulder that is weak or partially frozen in a way it isn't used to, and yes, a tear in one of the rotator cuff muscles can very likely occur. There are four muscles in the rotator cuff group, by the way. (I get many blank stares when I ask which rotator cuff muscle was torn.) These injuries can be easily prevented through regular exercise in which the shoulder joint is moved through its normal range of motion, thus saving patients the anguish, inconvenience and expense of a debilitating shoulder injury.

Yes, our joints need to move through their ranges of motion or else they will *literally* "glue" together. Once this happens, it can be quite a challenge to "unglue" them. There is a type of tissue in our body that is not talked about a lot, but it is starting to get more and more attention, as its importance is finally being recognized. It is called "fascia." We've all heard of muscles, tendons, and ligaments. These are primarily what is talked about when you hear the

90

term "soft tissues." You may not remember exactly what they are, but you probably recognize the names from a basic science class somewhere along the course of your education. Fascia, however, is also extremely important and is certainly NOT something that should be overlooked. "Fascia is a thin casing of connective tissue that surrounds and holds every organ, blood vessel, bone, nerve fiber and muscle in place. The tissue does more than provide internal structure; fascia has nerves that make it almost as sensitive as skin. When stressed, it tightens up." (Johns Hopkins: Muscle Pain: It May Actually Be Your Fascia)

Fascia is actually made up of collagen fibers and also acts as a sense organ by triggering changes in the body's chemistry in response to changes in the soft tissues. In some cases, there are less fibers and the fascia looks like cobwebs or spiderwebs. Over time, more and more fibers will grow and the fascia will get thick. Sometimes this is a good thing and sometimes it isn't. Thickening fascia can ultimately adhere muscles together or adhere muscles to bone and cause joints to not move properly, as in the case of the shoulder joint that I mentioned earlier. These are referred to as "adhesions" and can be the cause of chronic pain for some people. Fascia thickens when you don't move certain areas regularly, although in some cases, the opposite is true. Chronic stress on a muscle or joint from overuse can also cause the fascia to thicken. Think about those movies with the old houses that have been abandoned for years, and how the cobwebs grow and grow. Stretching and moving are the best ways to "clear the cobwebs out." Acupuncture is also really great for this as it loosens tight fibers. Below is a picture of what fascia looks like between the soft tissue layers.

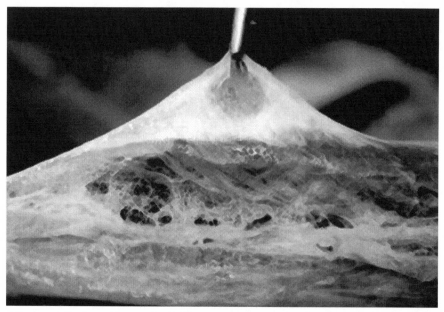

Photo credit: http://www.fascialfitness.net.au/articles/fascia-thickness-aging-and-flexibility/

If you get a chance, go on YouTube and search for "The Fuzz Speech." I had a chance to see this video when I was in Chinese Medicine school and I never forgot it. Disclaimer: this video contains footage of a human cadaver, so only watch it if you're not squeamish. If you don't want to watch, I'll tell you the basic premise. As I mentioned earlier, when we don't move our bodies regularly like they are designed to move, fascia actually grows between muscle layers and between muscles and bones. The less the area moves, the thicker the fascia gets. What eventually happens is that your muscles and joints are UNABLE to move ("glued" in place) even when you want to move them!

We focus a lot on the skeletal muscles when we think about exercise, but we don't think as much about the importance of exercise for the proper movement of our organs. Remember those "adhesions" I mentioned earlier? The fascia that can develop between muscle layers and between muscle and bone? Well, those same adhesions can develop around and in between your organs, as well, making them less able to perform their proper functions. Our organs require a certain amount of space to move, as many of them expand and contract, and adhesions can prevent this from happening. Moving your body through exercise also helps clear the cobwebs away from your organs too! Exercise is great for your heart, your lungs, your liver, kidneys and for your digestion system!

Exercise not only keeps your muscles, bones and organs moving freely, it also *strengthens* all the soft tissues in your body, your organs and your bones too. The BEST way to maintain bone density is to purposely and safely increase stress on your skeletal system through "weight-bearing" exercise. That means engaging in activities where you are on your feet, so that your skeletal system is bearing your weight. Walking, hiking, running, dancing... these activities are great for your lower half but don't forget about your upper half!! Yoga and strength training are really great for strengthening your upper body. Strengthening the muscles around your joints helps to keep your joints stable and less likely to deteriorate as you get older. Most of the joints in the body are surrounded by elastic-like muscles and tendons, which help to keep the bones joined together where they are supposed to be. When these muscles get tight, weak or deteriorate, they cannot hold the joint together properly and the joint will start malfunctioning.

Exercise is also great for mood regulation. Even just gentle exercise, like walking, hiking, yoga and tai chi can increase energy and calm anxiety. Maybe when you are feeling stressed, you try going out for a walk instead of reaching for that bottle of wine. It really DOES work. Walking outside (especially in the woods) is one of my most effective strategies for combating stress, anxiety and irritability. When I start to feel pent up, I try to get outside and walk. I always feel better when I get back. Getting outside, in general, is huge for me. Sometimes I feel like the walls of my house start to close in on me and I need to be soothed by wide open spaces.

Exercise is also **amazing** for the immune system. Not only does it strengthen your heart and your lungs, but it is *required* for proper functioning of your lymphatic system. The lymphatic system makes up a huge part of our immune system. It's a network of vessels throughout the body that transports fluid, and acts as our body's "sewerage" system. This means that it transports and eliminates toxic wastes from our body. Our lymphatic system relies on the contraction of our skeletal muscles to serve as an enormous pumping system that pumps waste from our body! In addition, our skeletal muscles also help pump blood in and out of them through the same squeezing mechanism. This is a huge help to our organs, especially the heart! So imagine how much happier the body is when you contract & relax (move) all its skeletal muscles in the form of exercise. This reduces stress on our organs and helps our bodies remove waste. This is huge!

The way I figure it is: You have to train for life. Exercise is a maintenance plan that is required to keep your body strong, mobile and agile, and it becomes even more important as we get older, because that is when our bodies become weaker, stiffer and more brittle. This is also when we tend to move *less*. We get "too busy" and we begin to prioritize other things over taking care of our bodies. We don't want to take the time or make the effort. We resist new experiences and trying something new. Don't let this happen to you!! Exercise can offset this and prolong this process. The more you move, the stronger and more flexible you will be, and the better the quality of life you will have moving forward. And you'll be far less prone to debilitating, accidental injuries. Yes, you might still slip in that icy parking lot, but your body will be able to handle it. You won't sustain an injury and have to make a trip to the ER.

Now, what kind of exercise you choose to do it up to you. There is no "one size fits all" here; this is extremely individual. Everyone has their own goals, interests, time constraints and availability options. At minimum, I recommend an exercise program consisting of some cardiovascular exercise (walking, hiking, running, biking, skiing, etc), coupled with joint mobility work (strength training, yoga, tai chi/martial arts). This way you are making sure to work your organs AND your joints. In light of all the things I talked about earlier, hopefully you can see how important it is to all *vary* your types of exercise. You want to engage in activities that allow you to go forwards, backwards, side to side, engage both upper and lower body and increase your heart rate some, so that you are getting all the possible benefits of exercise.

Like maintaining a healthy diet, you CANNOT underestimate the value of regular exercise when it comes to your health. MAKE TIME to maintain your body, I beg you! It's the only one you have and it needs to last many years. As a health care practitioner, I have seen countless women, who suffer from chronic pain, who I *know* would feel a lot better if they just took the time to keep their bodies in better working order. But they *don't* make the time.. and I don't know why! I realize that this sometimes feels like "work" (especially when you are first getting the exercise habit established), and I'm not going to lie.. sometimes it really is work. You'll not want to do it sometimes, but most times, you should DO IT ANYWAYS. When I am struggling for motivation on certain days, I tell myself: "I won't regret it if I do it, but I WILL regret it if I don't." And this is true. I have NEVER finished a workout and said "gee, I wish I didn't do that." But I HAVE, on many occasions, let a day slip by without getting a workout in and regretted that I didn't make time that day.

If you think you don't have time to workout, you probably just need to shift your priorities around a bit. Surely there is an activity you engage in for at least 30 minutes a day, that you can replace with a walk/run/hike, some yoga, tai chi/qi gong or strength training, and then maybe choose some more active options for when you have more free time: riding a bike, hiking, skiing, skating, dancing, longer yoga or strength training sessions. Get outside when you can! While I have my issues with smart watches, they can be helpful motivators for those who struggle to get enough exercise in, so use one of those if you think it's helpful.

It takes TIME and EFFORT to care for your body. There is no way around it. If you are constantly prioritizing other people's needs and wants (work, family, friends, etc) over taking care of your own body, then you cannot be surprised when your neglected body starts to complain. And it isn't going to get better just because you choose to ignore it. That isn't how this goes. YOU HAVE TO MAKE THE TIME.

Find a Group - Be Accountable

Another tool that is really helpful for many people is to find a friend or a group to exercise with. Accountability is a big motivator for MANY people who can't muster their own motivation. Usually planning to meet someone at a particular time for a particular activity gets most people out the door, when they may have stayed home otherwise. Because of this, there are many small, locally run clubs/groups in most areas for various disciplines: hiking, walking, running, cycling and then you can easily find some group classes for other activities, like yoga, strength training and tai chi/qi gong. There are typically more than most people realize.. I recommend just asking around. Talk to people that you know engage in these activities and see what they are doing and where. And remember: **everyone** was a beginner once, so beginners don't need to be ashamed or embarrassed of being a beginner. It's unfortunate... but I know they often are, and this poses a large roadblock to achieving *consistency*, which you NEED to get better and stronger. New things are always awkward and hard at first - this is why I wrote a whole section about getting out of your comfort zone. This is where you need to dig in and use that information. My tip: runners and hikers are *particularly* friendly to newcomers, and also know that *most* running groups also have walking groups for those who cannot or desire not to run. I recommend joining a friendly group of people who are meeting regularly to engage in exercise. You won't *just* be getting exercise, you will also be potentially connecting with people who have the same goals/interests, and this will give you new ideas and open new doors. If you don't like one group, look for another. I have been a member of a women's-only fitness group for years, but something I learned about myself along the way: I really enjoy the energy of men, too. So I prefer coed groups. But that's just me.

Tai Chi/Qi Gong (Special Mention)

I wanted to make particular mention of a very unique, but extremely beneficial form of exercise that originated in China and is still widely used in China. I'm sure you've probably heard of "tai chi" in some form or another. More people have heard of tai chi, but not qi gong. Tai chi, which originates from a defensive form of an ancient Chinese martial art, *is* qi gong. Tai chi is made up of very specific sets of exercises to create "forms". There are many different tai chi "forms". Qi gong is discrete exercises, while tai chi is the entire sequence. Qi gong is a train car; tai chi is the train. Make sense? I like to think of *qi gong* (which loosely translates to "energy work") as the Chinese version of yoga, which originated in India. Like yoga, qi gong combines movement and breath in an effort to move the "qi" (circulation) in particular parts of the body, depending on the exercise. Also like yoga, there are different "exercises" (or poses) for different parts of the body. Unlike yoga, all of the exercises are done standing (or there are seated variations for those who cannot stand for long periods of time). Qi gong exercises are typically much more gentle and consist of standing while engaging in slow and intentional movements of the upper body. These intentional movements are designed to take each body part through its full range of motion, slowly and gently, but effectively. You can get through a series of exercises that will move your entire body, in about 5-20 minutes a day. Qi gong is intended to be "weight bearing" for the purpose of strengthening the back and legs. If you are ever interested in investigating qi gong exercises, go to YouTube and search "qi gong". You will be amazed at what you find! While you can find in person training here in the US, it is not as widely available.

Qi gong is SO incredibly beneficial.. and yet.. very few people know anything about. I would like to see it gain more popularity, especially in the older populations. Doing 5 minutes of qi gong exercises or tai chi every day would literally be a game changer for so many people. In China, it is a common sight to see people gather in the parks and perform tai chi as a group. Most people would be too embarrassed in the US (at least where I live) to do tai chi in the park, fearful that people would point, look and judge. That is our culture.

We spend our lives fearing judgement by others and so we don't pursue the things we really want to. This is what we need to break out of, ladies!!!! *This* destructive pattern.

Yoga (Special Mention #2)

Most people think of yoga as stretching, and indeed it is. It is flexibility and mobility training, and it is VERY important because this type of training allows your body to get into its proper alignment. By stretching all of the muscles in your body regularly, your spine and your joints can function exactly how they are supposed to. We ALL get out of alignment because we create stress on our bodies by doing too much of one activity and not enough of others. Or maybe we are just born that way.. hardly anyone is actually symmetrical.. and then we make it worse by sitting too much, standing too much, running too much, typing too much.. who knows! But this is what happens. Yoga is a great way of getting your body back into balance. I am talking about gentle, recovery yoga here.. not hot, intense yoga!

Now, I am HUGELY guilty of skipping my flexibility training.. yoga, foam rolling, recovery type "exercise." I'll admit.. I'm kind of a spaz! Yoga means I have to stay mostly still and go slow, and if you have been skipping this type of training for awhile, it is downright painful! I don't like to stop moving for the sake of doing yoga. I come up with lots of great excuses to skip the stretching and rolling. I actually did a really great job of avoiding it throughout my Ironman training! Go me! No! BAD me!! Don't do this. Learn from my mistakes!

Yoga has now officially won a place in my heart and I have come to realize that of ALL the training that I do for my triathlons, yoga needs to be priority #1 and NOT priority #ONE MILLION.. and this is why. I started to experience ongoing low back/hip pain while training for my Ironman. Thankfully, it wasn't debilitating and I was able to continue training and completed the race successfully, but I started to have nagging, chronic pain. I thought it would go away after I completed the race and could rest and move my focus to more strength and flexibility training, but it didn't. Then I started to experience knee pain. Debilitating knee pain that made me stop running for the first time since I started running many years ago. So the nagging back and hip, and now the knee. This wasn't me. Sure, I've had my share of aches and pains, but never something that actually STOPPED me from training. I was becoming frustrated as I tried everything I could think of to do. I rested, I trained differently, I got massages, acupuncture, chiropractic.. at one point I even tried a liver cleanse - I thought that maybe I had some systemic inflammation going on.. nothing helped long term. I was worried that I was broken, never to be "normal" again. Then one of my patients mentioned yoga therapy, and I thought.. "that's the only thing I haven't tried!" And it turns out.. that's what actually "fixed" me (well, not quite yet, but I am on my way!).

As it turns out, I pounded my low back and pelvis right out of alignment during the hours I spent crammed onto a bike and running (DUH!).. and since I was doing ZERO flexibility training to help offset that during Ironman training... it's no wonder that I was all out of whack at the end of it all. Thankfully, I found a really great yoga therapist to help get me back on track. I have had to painfully stretch and roll my back, hips and legs to get everything back into better alignment, and only NOW, a year a half later, do I feel like I am making headway. And now I KNOW. Had I been doing all of that before, I wouldn't be struggling the way I am now. I will not make that mistake again! Mistakes like these are what trip us up with chronic pain and more severe injuries. It can be avoided! Don't skip the yoga! But I STILL have to force myself to do it... !

Part of the problem is that I am getting older. The older we get, the MORE we need this type of training. We have spent many years getting weaker and out of alignment and we NEED to keep our bodies in good working order.

I am thankful to have found this. I was honestly discouraged, like so many people are.. thinking they will never get better. You can get better.. you just need to find the right tools! Keep looking and don't stop trying to get better! Never give up!

SO now.. I'm a yoga fan! It has connected me with my body in a way that many other forms of exercise haven't.

Don't Forget About Sleep

Ahhhh.. the last section in this part, but certainly NOT the least. Sleep. I've no doubt that you know in your mind that sleep is important, but let me just share some additional information on just how important it really is.

In Chinese medicine, there is something called the "qi cycle," or the "qi clock." The theory is that each organ system in the body is most active during the same 2 hour block every day, working on our 24 hour clock system. You can take a look at the diagram below to see which organ systems are active at the different times during the day.

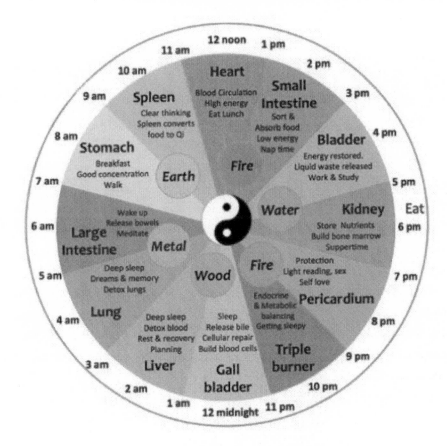

I would like to bring your attention specifically to the gallbladder, liver and lung in the lower left corner. These 3 organ systems are most active at *night* and maintenance of these organs require you to be RESTING, preferably sleeping! This is essentially when your body runs its "cleaning" cycle. Your liver and your lungs work together to cleanse your blood while you are resting. It's hard to do maintenance on moving parts, right? This is the time your body needs to close for maintenance! Because of this clock, it is HIGHLY recommended and beneficial for your body if you can arrange to get to sleep before 11:00 PM. It is also helpful if you can avoid using any substances before bed that hinder liver function.. like medications and alcohol... OI! I know that is a tall order for many! I KNOW that MANY women struggle with sleep issues. This is really what is BEST for your liver, and also.. believe it or not, will improve the quality of your sleep and recovery. Alcohol and medications, while they may help you fall asleep, actually interfere with your body's ability to **truly** rest and recover. So you may *sleep*, but your body cannot fully complete what needs to be done. Your sleep quality will be hindered, so you make wake not feeling rested or suffer from fatigue during the daytime. I know that might be overwhelming - I'm just here to give you the facts! There are other ways to improve sleep without turning to therapies that damage the liver.

You can also take a peek at the section between 1pm and 3pm.. NAP TIME!! I don't know about you, but this is the time of day when I always feel like I need a nap. When I get the opportunity, I will lie down and rest for 20-30 minutes. I'm not much of a "napper" so I may just doze off for a few minutes, or not at all, but just lying down quietly, taking a little "reset" (have you ever noticed how close "rest" and "reset" are? Same, same!) helps tremendously. Since I get to make my own work schedule, I have even started to block off the 1-3pm time frame on my long work days so I can recharge, and be my best. Who wants to be taken care of by a tired and strung out health care provider??? My patients definitely appreciate my energy to care for them into the evening hours. I realize that not many people have the time and place to be able to pull off a midday "reset," but if there is any way at all that you can make this happen, even just for a few minutes, it will help your physical and mental health. I do wish that culturally, we would see the importance of an afternoon rest time and incorporate one into school and work days. Some countries already do this (Spain is one I know for sure) and that is because it really helps productivity! We would be MUCH happier people. And healthier, too.

Dealing With The "I Can't Sleep" Anxiety

You've been there, right? You can't sleep so you start to feel anxious about not sleeping because you have a million things to do tomorrow and how are you going to do all these things when you don't get any sleep?!?! You keep watching numbers on the clock by. Then you get yourself all worked up, which pretty much GUARANTEES that you are not going to sleep any time soon! I have been there!

My advice for these situations is that you HAVE to try to relax. It is *normal* to be unable to sleep sometimes. Everyone I know has issues on occasion, whether it is situational stress, location, premenstrual/menopausal, seasonal, or maybe it's something you did differently that day that you don't normally do. Most of us can function just fine on little to no sleep, in the short term. If you are normally a decent sleeper (meaning: you don't need substance assistance to sleep), and you start experiencing bouts of sleeplessness, know that it is likely only temporary and it will pass, and you will get by just fine. Remember that getting yourself all worked up over it only makes it worse. If it lasts more than a week or two, I would start doing some investigation on possible causes. Trying to figure out the cause is necessary for determining the treatment. If you feel all worked up, you can try some things to help calm you. Read a book, listen to calming music, stories or meditations (there are great apps for that), have a cup of tea (I love the Yogi Bedtime tea). Maybe these things will help, maybe they won't, but staying calm is going to give you a much better chance of resting than to lie in bed with your heart pounding out of your chest.

Suggestions For Improving Sleep

There are many reasons why sleep can be an issue for many women. My suggestions are to take a look and try a few of these ideas before you turn to "stronger" methods of treatment. The reason you are not sleeping well could very well be something that you can change. If it's something you can take away, then that is better than adding something new!

Take a look at your caffeine intake.

Caffeine interferes with sleep and some women are more sensitive to it than others. And honestly, your body can decide at any time that it's "sensitive" to it. A few years ago, I started having issues falling asleep at night. It seemed to happen fairly suddenly and it persisted. It took me some time to figure out that it was the afternoon tea or coffee that I was drinking. Although I was drinking it around 3pm and attempting to go to bed around 10pm, my body was still reacting to it at that time, and through the night. Information about caffeine states that it should be out of my system by then. But clearly not since my system was still amped up. Through some of my own experimenting, I discovered that I can drink caffeine in the afternoons in the winter, but I cannot in the summer. Summertime makes my body more sensitive to the caffeine. In Chinese medicine, caffeine generates "heat" internally. So it makes sense that the stimulating effect would be exaggerated in the summer. So I have to be careful. I recommend taking a look at your own intake if you are having issues sleeping. Are you drinking anything with caffeine in it in it after 12pm? Coffee, tea, sodas, energy drinks, even some protein shakes/diet supplements can contain "green tea extract." Kombucha, which I am a HUGE fan of, is made from fermented tea. It has small amounts of caffeine, and even that will mess with my sleep. (As a side note, I also discovered that coffee worsens my anxiety symptoms, so I no longer drink coffee either.)

Take a look at your medications.

There are actually a number of medications that cause sleeplessness as one of the their main side effects. Your doctor may not have informed you about it, and most people don't read the medication inserts (but they should!). You may not even know that something you are taking is causing your issues. The biggest culprits are:

- Anti-depressants

- Decongestants (like Sudafed)
- Stimulants (like Ritalin)
- Corticosteroids (like prednisone)
- Beta blockers (for blood pressure regulation)
- ACE Inhibitors (also for blood pressure regulation)
- Statins (for lowering cholesterol)
- Thyroid hormone replacement (like levothyroxin)
- Theophylline (in medications that treat asthma)

There are others too, so I would check the side effects of ANY drug you are taking regularly, whether it is over the counter or prescription. If you decide to make changes, discuss them with your pharmacist or doctor. In some cases, it is not advisable to suddenly discontinue use, so you and your doctor should work together to change your meds or wean you off your current ones.

Get to sleep before 11:00PM.

As I mentioned earlier, you will get a better night's sleep if you can get to bed and be asleep before 11pm. One your body goes into "liver" time, it may be harder to fall asleep if you aren't already. Then you may miss your window and not actually get to sleep until much later. Your body needs this time to recover and recharge.

Avoid heavy meals before bed.

Eating later is fine. Some people find that they cannot rest if they are hungry (me!!). But you don't want to eat a super heavy, fatty, greasy, restaurant meal before bed, if you can help it. If you bombard your digestive system with too much work right before you intend on resting, it will be too busy trying to deal with the barrage of food to be able to rest, and it will keep you up!

Adjust the temperature where you are sleeping.

Room temperature can interfere with sleep, especially heat. Our bodies actually need to be a bit cooler for proper rest. As a premenopausal women, I can definitely attest to the fact that heat and sleep are not buddies. Last summer I experienced insomnia for the entire month of August. It had been a hot and sunny summer and it just got to the point where my body temperature was too elevated to be able to sleep. I actually didn't start sleeping normally again until fall rolled in and the temperatures dropped. Just like that, like a switch, I was sleeping normally again.

Note where you are in your menstrual cycle. Or if you are in menopause.

Our body temperatures elevate a bit between ovulation and menses. Pre-menstrual sleep disruptions and night sweats are common. If your sleep issues are due to hormonal fluctuations, they will likely pass once the hormones re-regulate. If your lack of sleep is becoming a problem and the hormones are not regulating, consider seeking out more *natural* therapies that help rebalance hormones (again: diet, exercise, yoga/meditation, Chinese medicine (acupuncture), herbal supplementation). If you are menopausal and your sleep is suffering, it's because your hormones are off-balance. These therapies will help you too! Sometimes the imbalance is just temporary while your body is "figuring it out." Sometimes it becomes more long term, and in which case, you should **work** to *rebalance* them. If you don't, it may not get better. Medications typically don't help your body rebalance, they just ADD whatever you might be missing. So when you stop taking the medications, you will still have problem.

Try calming routines before bed.

If you are having trouble falling asleep because you feel "amped" up (and you have already checked your caffeine and medication intake), avoid any activities that might make you feel stressed (TV programs with emotional subject matter or social media) and instead turn to activities that make you feel calmer, like reading, meditating, yoga. As I mentioned earlier, there are some great phone apps with meditations on them. You can pop in some earbuds and listen. White noise can be helpful if you are a "light" sleeper. We sleep year-round with a fan on in my house!

Try some gentle supplements.

Bedtime teas are great. You can get those at most supermarkets. I mentioned tart cherry juice (or concentrate) earlier. Tart cherry juice has naturally occurring melatonin that can help regulate melatonin in the body. Tart cherry juice and plain greek yogurt make an awesome bedtime snack, as you get the protein and the calming cherry juice. Magnesium supplementation can be helpful too. Find a good magnesium supplement and take before bed. Melatonin can be helpful but it is severely OVERUSED. Melatonin supplements are **not** meant for long term use, as this will lead to reduction in the body's own production of it. This will cause a rebound effect. If you are having trouble sleeping, you can also try small doses of melatonin, but YOU SHOULD NOT STAY ON IT. A few days to a week, tops. Then you should discontinue use. When it comes to other supplements, I recommend consulting with someone trained in prescribing herbal supplements. Herbal supplements have to properly matched with the actual cause of your sleep issues in order for them to be effective. There's no "one size fits all" with herbs, and you can do damage if you take them improperly. They are very specific, and so you should speak with someone who knows about them.

Chances are, some of these things are going to help you. If you try a bunch of things yourself and you still can't get to the bottom of your issues, find a trained professional who can help you. Acupuncture is VERY effective at treating sleep issues, so seek out an acupuncturist. It is my advice to you that you exhaust every possible avenue before turning to medications. You have to figure out the WHY, so you can figure out the HOW. Don't give up! It's only temporary and it WILL get better if you work at it. Now go get some rest! You probably need it!

III

Women's Mental & Emotional Health

Why Mental Health is Just As Important As Physical Health

When many people think of "health and wellness," especially people in our traditional medical community, they don't often give mental health the attention that they give our *physical* health. When you go for a standard check-up, do you get a mental health evaluation? Does anyone ask you about your stress level? Whether you are feeling depressed? Anxious? Happy? Do you feel like no one really cares how you *feel* on the inside, only how you on the outside? If you do, you are certainly not alone in that.

I am not entirely sure why the mental health aspect of our bodies has been so neglected. Although, I can make a guess, if you are interested! Me, having the curious mind that I do, I am always searching for the *whys* in everything. So here goes. Once upon a time, there lived a French philosopher named Rene Descartes. Ever heard of him? "Rene Descartes (1596-1650) was a brilliant philosopher, mathematician, and scientist. Most scholars consider him responsible for modern medicine's splitting the mind and mental issues away from the body and its diseases. As a result, the mind and its mental disorders became the province of the 17th century church while medicine and science focused on the body and its diseases to lead a new scientific revolution." (Smith, 2018). Descartes played a huge role in modern medicine's focus on physical disease, and as a sad result, mental health issues go largely ignored by Western medical practitioners. Ironically, most of the mental health care that patients receive is from their medical doctors, who actually get very little training in this field! Their "care" comes mostly in the form of medication prescriptions or referrals to practitioners who are better trained in this area (hopefully!).

This is another reason why I love Chinese medicine and its treatment of the mind-body connection. Ancient Chinese philosophy is devoid of that split. In fact, in Chinese medicine theory, each organ system is ascribed a corresponding emotion. For example, sadness is associated with the lung. Intense or prolonged grief can indeed damage the lungs and conversely, chronic lung issues can make a person more susceptible to experiencing sadness and grief. Prolonged periods of stress affects liver function. It is not uncommon at all for stress to exacerbate many health conditions, like pain, digestive issues, menstrual issues and headaches/migraines, and for chronic, unmanaged stress to lead to more serious and chronic health issues, like cancer.

Declining kidney function is associated with increased fear. Have you ever wondered why we tend to become more fearful as we get older? According to Chinese medicine, it is due to the aging of our kidneys. Our adrenal glands are actually physically located on top of our kidneys. Obviously, our adrenal glands make adrenaline, which is one of the hormones produced when we feel fear. The glands also produce cortisol, our "fight-or-flight", or "stress" hormone (which we've all heard so much about). The proximity of the adrenal glands to the kidneys means that the kidneys are largely affected by, and directly responsible for immediately processing hormonal changes from the adrenal glands. If the kidneys can't do their job properly, this will cause an imbalance in the adrenals. Conversely, an imbalance in the adrenals will cause the kidneys to work harder. When the adrenal glands work too hard for too long, they get tired out! This is what we call "adrenal fatigue" or "adrenal insufficiency." The adrenal glands are super important, and their function impacts many other important functions in your body, like your liver and your heart. So you tell me... can chronic anxiety, stress, and fear impact your health?! Absolutely!!!! It's a no brainer!

So, in the previous section, we talked about diet, menstrual health, exercise and physical rest which, while these also will have some impact on your mental health, they will not fix mental discomfort caused by lifestyle, trauma or problematic thought patterns. Those things will help your body better *cope* with the effects of the uncomfortable emotions, but they will not treat the root if the "root" is, in fact, based in your mental and emotional health. You *need* to ultimately treat the cause(s) of your issues. Depending on your history and your age, this could be quite a task.. and for many, emotional discomfort can be far more intense and painful than physical discomfort. But if you truly want to heal, truly want to make sure your body is as nourished as it can be, you HAVE to recognize the role that your emotional and mental self play into your day to day lives. You can **not** afford to ignore it.

Mental Health and Women in Modern Society

"To be nobody but yourself —
in a world which is doing its best, night and day, to make you everybody
else — means to fight the hardest battle which any human being can
fight;
and never stop fighting."
- ee cummings

This has been said a million times in a million different places, and I am going to say it again. It is HARD to be a nourished woman in today's modern society. The demands that are placed upon us are a huge burden to bear. The worst part is that WE are our own worst enemies, and I am not just talking about the pressure put on us by other women (which is high), I am also talking about the pressure we put on *ourselves*, which is even higher! We take on so many outside responsibilities that we neglect ourselves for lack of time and resources, and many are raised to believe that this is what we are "supposed to" do, what *women* do, as wives and mothers. According to whom? Whose rules are these? I mean, who decided that we, as women, are to be born to give and give, to take nothing for ourselves, then to shrivel up and die? Is this not what is expected of women in our society? I ask myself these questions often when I feel a case of the "supposed-tos" coming on. I ask myself, "Says who?" Not me!!! I didn't make those rules! And neither did you. So you are not obligated to live by them. Now you know that. But really convincing yourself and changing the dialogue in your own head is the *hard* part.

As women desiring to be our own selves, we get caught in the "in between." Many of us want careers and lives of our own, but we also desire the family unit: marriage, kids, the big house, the "American Dream." Then we are also typically the first ones to let our own needs, wants and careers go to the wayside so that we can be the caretakers of the family and family dwelling. I'm not sure that we are programmed to do that - I know that some people believe it is nurture vs. nature. I personally think that as women, we are caretakers by nature and that many of us *instinctively* want to take care of others above ourselves, especially those we love. We are excellent multitaskers for a reason. I have spent much time poking around inside my own head over this issue, and I truly believe, in my own case, that it is just how I am wired.

Back to the issue of "wanting it all." There are two major drawbacks here to "having it all," time and energy. If you are a woman with a career and family, you have probably already learned that EACH of those is *more* than a full-time job. Now you are trying to put them both together. Although careers *can* be part-time, they rarely are. If you are not in control of your own schedule, then you are probably working more than you want to be. Obviously, the "standard" American work week is 40 hours. In some cases, this is the low end. In most cases, employees have to work a minimum of 32 hours a week before they even qualify for benefits such as health insurance and retirement plans. Couple that with the fact that it is the expectation of the American nuclear family unit that the parents are the #1 caretakers of the children, typically with the women taking a majority of the load, and you can already see that there is simply not enough room in one's life to work full-time, take care of a family AND oneself. Most women are doing the first two and neglecting the last one. And therein lies the problem. Years and years of giving to others, and not taking the time to nourish their own bodies takes quite a toll on women, as you can imagine. Then they show up in my office with issues that will likely take months to years to fully treat. Depending on how long they've been "running on fumes," they may *never* be able to recover.

Nourishing yourself: eating healthfully, exercising and resting properly... takes up a good chunk of time. If you're engaging in physical or mental maintenance practices, like massage, acupuncture, meditation, group workouts or classes, or just heading out for activities you enjoy - this is a great thing - but it does require one thing that many women don't have. Time. And it's no wonder! We're all trying to be superheroes. We're not superheroes. We're just human beings, trying to do our best here!

The expectations for women in our society are oppressive. We are suffocating underneath them! I see it every single day in my practice. We all know that time is limited. "Never enough time in a day" is a common saying, right? Let me say this with a running metaphor: if you want longevity, to finish the marathon of life and in the best possible shape, you **NEED** to slow your pace. If you sprint, rush through, you will burn out, not make it or limp to the end. Which one do you prefer? Would you rather have slower, more enjoyable days on a daily basis or work like a dog for weeks, maybe months, years on end, looking forward to that vacation, or I dare say.. retirement? I am blown away by people who work for years and years, never rest or take vacation, all because they are working towards retirement.. and then they get there (IF they get there) and are wholly unfulfilled because they have no idea how to enjoy it, or worse yet, they are *unable* to enjoy it because they are unwell after spending years not taking care of themselves. Or, in cases such as my dad's, die before you even fully make it there. This makes me sad.

The time to start taking care of yourself if RIGHT NOW. You have my permission, now give yourself permission too!

Sure, there's hardly a time when we don't feel like we have a million things to do and we are expected to do more than most of us are actually physically, mentally and emotionally capable of... but YOU can slow it down. You can shift your thought patterns. You can say NO. YOU can decide what your life looks like and only *you* can make that happen. You'll probably have to make some changes, and no, it might not be easy. But no one else will ever do that for you. You *should* make that happen, and not only because *you're* worth it. But because our daughters and their daughters are worth it, too. If you have sons, you can help shape their expectations too, so that women can believe that taking care of themselves is important. Like it or not, we are the caretakers of the world. What would the world be like without our loving and nurturing women?

I Don't "Have" To - I "Choose" To

One thing that has really helped me deal with the not-so-pleasant aspects of daily living is to fully understand that most things in life are a *choice.* Don't get me wrong, I understand that things happen that are NOT a choice... but for the most part, we *choose* how to spend our time, and our life. From the small, trivial stuff, like laundry to the larger ones, like careers and partners. We are never really "stuck." We may feel like we are. We may not like the other choices when it comes to making changes, but for the most part, we do have **choices**.

And this is an important thing for me to know because it staves off the resentment, for one. As I am folding endless amounts of laundry or spending yet another evening preparing dinner in the kitchen, I may be frustrated. Then I remind myself that my small, nuclear family is my #1 priority in life, and that I do all the laundry because I *choose* to. I cook healthy meals because I *choose* to. I could tell my family members that they could do their own laundry, and we could eat out all the time like many other people. I don't prefer those choices, and so I continue to make mine every day. I do all the laundry, I shop, I prepare, I cook. Sometimes I don't want to clean up and so I make the choice to leave dishes until the next day. Could someone else clean up? Probably. But they don't make that choice, and I know it, and I am not responsible for other people's choices. So it's clean up or leave it. I am tired at the end of the day, so I am much happier doing dishes in the morning.

As far as the bigger things go... these choices obviously have a much larger impact on your life. You hate your job or your career? Change it. Yes, it is that simple. No, it might not be *easy..* but it is not complicated. Investigate your other choices. You could choose to quit on the spot and be unemployed. Then maybe you won't have income coming in that you prefer to have. Obviously you are *choosing* to go to a job you hate over losing that income, and the impacts that this may have. So, whether you realize it or not, you are STILL making a choice to go to work every day and you have decided that going to work every day is the better choice for you. So own up to that. Maybe you are in an awful marriage, but you feel like you "can't" leave for various reasons. Remind yourself that you CAN leave, you just choose *not* to because of reasons X, Y and Z.

I started to change my own dialogue around a lot of things. I no longer say "I have to," unless I truly do, like in the case of biological needs. Now I say "I choose to." My 5th grade teacher would be proud, as I also no longer say "I can't," rather "I can, but I *choose* not to." It really does make a difference. Then instead of feeling powerless and out of control, you realize that you are *powerful* and in *full* control of the experience of your life.

When it comes to other people, on the other hand... it is wise to understand that you *cannot* control other people and their choices. This is definitely an appropriate case of the "can'ts". It will behoove you to accept and understand that you are not responsible for the choices of others, and you *can't* force others to make the choices the way you would make them. They are not you. As Morgan Freeman clearly states in the movie "Bruce Almighty", "You can't mess with free will." You are, however, responsible for your own choices and for how you respond to and treat others. I believe that fully understanding this concept decreases frustration towards others by A LOT, and decreasing frustration will make YOU a much happier person, and probably those you maintain relationships with. I tell my daughter this often, because I wish I had fully known it for the first 30 years of my life. It is very freeing.

This is an area that mental health counseling really helped me with. I learned that by being empathetic towards others' struggles, trying to figure out what their struggles are, while also setting myself apart from it and realizing that *their* issues are not MY issues, allowed me not to take other people's "issues" personally. In this way, you can choose how to respond to someone else's struggles or negativity. Emotionally stepping outside the box and looking in, means that you can exercise your choice to choose whether or not you want to engage, be offended or ignore. Personally, I am very sensitive to the emotions of others around me, especially when it comes to certain people in my life. Recognizing that fact gives me the power to choose whether or not I want to let that energy inside of me.

Knowing that you are actually in control of your own life, and not just a "victim" of circumstance, is really empowering and can entirely transform parts of your life. That's why I mentioned it. It seems like a simple concept, but sometimes it's the small shifts in thinking that create the largest ripples.

Striving For Balance: Chasing The Wild Goose

How do you balance living each day to its fullest, while also planning for longevity? Any moment, our lives could be cut short. We all know people that this has happened to. Or we might live to a ripe old age and in which case, we probably want to be as healthy and happy as possible while we get there. So while we might want to live as though every day is our last (at least I do!), we also need to live with the knowledge that more than likely, unless we are terminally ill or doing something extremely dangerous, we are more likely to live another day. We'll probably a long string of more days. So how do we fully enjoy life while not completely sabotaging our family, our work, our health, or our mental and emotional well being? That is really the key to finding "balance."

Most days I think that concept is a pipe dream. A mirage. A wild goose chase. This is probably the biggest struggle of my modern life, and while yes, I do recognize the fact that I am very fortunate to have this be my biggest problem in life, I am pretty sure I've caused myself much mental and emotional strife trying to achieve it. Until I finally realized that it's actually unattainable, at least on a long term basis. Don't get me wrong, I can attain it for a few days.. maybe a few weeks.. that might be pushing it. But come that last week of my menstrual cycle, and... FUGETABOUTIT! Last week I was content working only 3 days, filling my other days with writing, working out and the mundane home maintenance tasks, but this week I hate my life, everyone is driving me crazy and I need to just pack my bags and move to a small village in a country in the middle of nowhere.

I've experimented a lot with trying to achieve balance, probably more than the average woman. I am not afraid to make changes, even drastic ones, in the name of this quest. After my daughter was born, I quit a very well-paying corporate career as a software engineer because I found that I was spending too much time working at a job that I felt was unfulfilling, and not enough time being available to the tiny person I just brought into the world. I wasn't OK with making her someone else's responsibility. So began my mission for work-life balance. I quit my job and went back to school to pursue a career in Chinese medicine. Why? Three reasons: 1: health and healing were definitely something I was way more excited about (and still am, obviously!) than software engineering, 2: I knew I could set up my own practice, be my own boss and make my own schedule, and 3: It was the most accessible career, practicality-wise, to my life as a mom who did not want to be away from her daughter for extended periods of time. Then my marriage ended. So, while I was working on building my practice as a single mom, I worked too little and was broke... but I did get to be available for my daughter, which was great. For quite while, I had more time than money. Eventually (years??), it seemed to stop tipping so far in either direction and has evened out a bit, but the scales still rock back and forth regularly. I'm still searching 13 years later, although I have most definitely gotten a lot closer. But still.. it's always too much or not enough of SOMETHING. Then when I think I've gotten my house of cards all set up, something out of my control comes and knocks them all down. Like a teenager with her own plans. Or my husband with his. A college that decides to discontinue its acupuncture program and let all of their faculty go (my part time stint as a college professor, which took me YEARS to procure). A pandemic!!!! Have you ever noticed that every time you finally manage to get money saved up, something happens and bye-bye savings? I honestly don't think the universe is conspiring against us. It is just *reminding* us how nonsensical our expectations really are. Hence is the quest for balance. The fact of the matter is, folks, we have so much less control of this so-called "balance" than we think we do. I so believe it's worth the work to get as close to it as you can. To sneak up on it, and maybe you can throw a blanket over its head, pin it down and wrangle it in. Or maybe not. But just keep in mind that it's elusive, and you will probably never catch it.

I know it's cliche, but it really is the journey that counts. So do me a favor, and don't make "balance" your end goal. If you cling to it too tightly, you will be frustrated when it disappears again, when "life" happens again. Change is inevitable. Life is like rowing your boat down the stream.. you never know what you are going to get. Sometimes the current is wild and crazy, and sometimes it's slow and steady and easy. Think about what "balance" means to you, visualize it and head towards it, but also be OK with changing course when needed.

Get In The Driver's Seat

*"**The first place we lose the battle is in our own thinking**.*
If you think it is permanent, then it's permanent.
If you think you've reached your limit, then you have.
If you think you will never get well, then you won't.
You have to change your thinking.
You need to see everything that's holding you back, every obstacle,
*every limitation as **only temporary**."*
- Joel Osteen

I wrote some of this book while camped out in the back of a vehicle during my daughter's lacrosse practices. I've spent countless hours driving to and watching her practice and compete in various sports over the years, beginning with gymnastics when she was six years old. I wasn't too excited about her newest passion. Lacrosse. Not really my favorite. She and her dad decided that she would sign up for travel lacrosse during a pandemic. Not only was I now required to drive her to practices a couple time a week (which were 30-40 minutes away from home) and travel out of town for tournaments, but I would also be unable to watch her practice due to do the "CoVid" pandemic, so I would need to find something to occupy me during her 90 minute practices. The whole lacrosse club thing was kinda sprung on me. I didn't choose it, and I wasn't too happy about it. I quietly fought it for a bit, but then I gave into it. This is where I brought in my "choose tos". I chose (and continue to choose) to be supportive of my daughter's goals of being a good lacrosse player, and so I made lemonade with my lemons! I decided to use the time to write.

We certainly find ourselves in situations that we might not like. Maybe the situation was forced on us, or maybe we made a wrong choice somewhere along the way. In any case, it happens to us all. But just because we end up in a less than desirable situation doesn't mean that we have to STAY in that situation forever. We have help, tools and choices available to us that we can use to drive change.

When I first became a mom, I struggled. I really didn't like being the mother of an infant. Or a toddler, really. Don't get me wrong, I love my daughter in a way that I would never have known was possible without her in my life. It was the stress of that very love and her dependence on me that made mothering such a tiny person so overwhelming and stressful. I grew up an independent, only child and being "needed" was never something I was used to. Keeping her healthy, safe, while also encouraging and allowing her to find her own inner peace was (and still can be) such an intense responsibility for me to bear. It is also one I take extremely seriously. I think early on, I resented and became overwhelmed by my own need to always put her first. I still wanted to do my own things, reach my own goals, go where I wanted to when I wanted to. But I also felt this intense NEED to put this tiny person first, that it was my duty to produce the best human being I possibly could. I think at time I thought I would NEVER get my independence back.

My whole life start to implode not long after my daughter was born. I realized that I hated my career choice and then later, my husband choice, and for the first time in my life, I think I knew what it felt like to be "depressed." All while dealing with a tiny (and very needy) child. I cried regularly. UGH. Things seemed scary and hopeless. Even so, I knew this was not acceptable to me. I knew I could do better. I wasn't OK with just remaining unhappy. I wanted to change it. I needed to change it.

And so change it, I did. All of it. (Except my daughter! I decided to keep her. HA HA.) Turns out... I am actually *good* at engineering (my first career choice) when it mattered to me... because over the next 10 years, I slowly re-engineered my entire life. I went back to school. I got a divorce (while in school!). I started a business. I got remarried. I took a teaching job. I wrote a book. These were all scary, too, but they were a GOOD kind of scary. A *necessary* kind of scary. I am thankful every day that I didn't just stay put where I was.

You can drive the change or the change can drive you. Some people are made so uncomfortable by change that they try resist it at all costs, even if it's in their best interest. If you are letting the change drive you, you might not like where it's taking you. If you are someone who feels like "bad" things always seem to happen to you, it may because you resist making scary (but necessary) changes, and so things change FOR you, but maybe not in the way you would have liked. For example, before my husband and I got together, he spent many years in an unhappy marriage. 16 years actually. He recalls that on many occasions, he was suspicious that his ex-wife was cheating on him. Yet, he buried his head in the sand and continued on without making any changes. Then one day, he actually caught her. The marriage ended. He was devastated over it and he spent *years* being angry and resentful and, sadly, so did his children. He actually has a similar story about the job he despised but stayed at for far too long. Things could have gone a lot smoother had the change been initiated beforehand, before the universe took control of it. And it will if you let it. So I recommend getting in the driver's seat. Just putting your intention and energy into solving a problem will cause things to begin to shift. You can do hard and scary things! You have no idea what you are capable of until you truly try!

I'm almost 45 now, and so I am able to look back at the different stages of my life. One thing I have definitely learned is that the phases of our lives are so transient. I've gotten through and done things that I didn't think were possible. One thing you can count on is that nothing ever stays the same, yet we often get wrapped up in our moment(s) of suffering and somehow think that we are going to suffer FOREVER. We don't have to!! If you get stuck in this thinking, then you WILL suffer forever. It is HUGELY important that you recognize this concept of *impermanence*. Maybe you are unhappy now, in your current situation. Maybe you don't feel good physically, are in pain or have been feeling anxious and unsettled. One thing you have to KNOW, absolutely *know* and be confident of is that this current state doesn't have to last. You can change it. If you don't know how to change it or make it better, look around you and seek people who can help you change it or make it better. And most importantly, BE OPEN to changing and trying new things. If you think you want to change, but you shoot down all suggestions, then you are resisting. If you are struggling with a health condition and you insist that you want it to get better, but you refuse to make dietary changes.. then you are actually *stopping* change from happening and telling the universe that you don't really want things to change. So you can't blame anyone but yourself when your condition doesn't improve..

Or maybe you really *are* in a situation that you cannot or will not change, as in the case of motherhood. Most of us aren't willing to give up our children and we don't aspire to be bad parents. But what you CAN change is your thinking. Your attitude. Children grow up and they do it fast, and many of us will still have a lifetime to live after they are grown. I choose to be the best parent I can be, and that means I have to sacrifice my own wants sometimes, but it is a sacrifice born out of love.

The worst thing you can do is to give up and give in.

Never give up hope and never stop trying!

Stop Ruminating & Just DO It

Oh my... as women, aren't we just the *queens* of rumination? The process of continuously thinking about the same thoughts, which tend to be sad or dark, is called **rumination**. It's pretty much the same as obsessing. Rumination is not productive. At all. It creates negative feelings for no reason whatsoever. It serves only to make you feel sad, worry or feel anxious or depressed. FOR NO REASON. Sometimes I swear my being WANTS to be anxious. Like, I literally force myself to stop thinking of one terrible thing that is making me anxious just to find myself thinking about a totally different one a few minutes later. (This does appear to be menstrual-cycle related.) It seems to be even worse when you are a mother, thinking about all the horrible (and highly unlikely, by the way!) things that could happen to you or your child. It's awful. And normal. The only way to keep it from getting under your skin is to accept what is happening and redirect your thoughts. Or distract yourself by turning your attention elsewhere.

No one really knows why we do this. I wish I did, so I could make it stop!! Women with certain personality types, perfectionists and those with a history of trauma tend to ruminate more than others. Sometimes I think I am searching for a way to control or be prepared for certain situations that probably won't even happen... Maybe it's the control freak in us. I am definitely in this group, and if you are too, this advice might benefit you.

Sometimes we just ruminate over issues for which we have no control. Other times, we ruminate about a situation for which we have control, worrying over all the possible outcomes of this decision we want to make. The most important thing you can do when it comes to dealing with these annoying, unproductive thoughts is to raise your level of self-awareness and pay attention to what is happening. Ask yourself whether your thoughts are actually of benefit to you in some way. Are you working on solving a problem? Are you searching for solutions? Can you actually change the outcome or control the situations you are worrying about? How likely is the situation you are thinking about even to happen? Now, if you are actually solving a real problem and your thoughts are in fact, helping you, then this is *problem-solving*, not rumination. These are productive thought processes. As I mentioned before, rumination is NOT productive.

Ruminating can be a major roadblock to reaching our goals. Maybe something inside of you really wants to run a 5k someday or.. better yet... open your own business! But every time you start thinking about this "thing" you want to do, your mind starts heading down every negative rabbit hole it can find, which does nothing except fill you with self-doubt. And then you talk yourself out of it. Yet again. What if, instead of letting your mind talk yourself out of these awesome ideas you have, you tell that ruminating mind to SHUT UP and you take action. You make a different decision this time. You register yourself for your first 5k. Or you take that first step to opening your own business, whatever that may be. You get the ball rolling!! You don't have to worry about what comes next, just TAKE THAT FIRST STEP. All it takes is **one** decisive moment to completely change your course, and this could very well be it. I decided to do a full Ironman triathlon by just clicking the "register" button. No way was I going to waste $600! I decided to change my career when I showed up for that college open house.

Do you have the ability to predict the future? If you are always worrying about the future and what happens in it, then that means you think you can control it.. can we really *control* the future? If you are always worrying about the past, then that means you think you can change it. Can we really *change* the past? No. We can't do either. We can only control the decisions we make in the present. So tell that mind to be quiet and make those decisions that make your soul happy instead! Our entire lives are made up of a long string of simple decisions. Left or right? You decide.

Follow your "Gut"

*"**Intuition**..*
When you don't know...
How you know...
But you know you know...
and you know you knew...
and that's all
you needed to know....."
-Unknown

S peaking of the soul... I wholly believe that we have this "voice" or "knowing" (as Glennon Doyle calls it in her book "Untamed") or "intuition" inside of us that guides us, that tells us what to do and what we *should* do. Many people call it different names, but all of us who live by it know it's there. But we have to listen, and we have to know how to hear it.

When I was growing up, my mom would make decisions based on her "gut instinct." "I just know," she would say. As a child and teenager, that would frustrate me as I couldn't rationalize or argue with that logic! I don't remember the exact time during my own development that I started to hear my own inner voice, but at some point I started recognizing that very "gut instinct" that my mother referred to. I remember it becoming really strong during my pregnancy with my daughter and it remains strong today. My pregnancy is when I *really* started to " go against the grain" and question common parenting practices. Up until that point, I pretty much did what I was "supposed" to do. I was the model American child and young adult. I grew up, went to school, got good grades, stayed out of trouble, went to college, got a "good" job, paid my taxes, got married, bought a house (oops, I think I did the last two in reverse!), had a child.... and then.... and THEN..... this inner voice emerged that started questioning EVERYTHING. I became the "crunchy" mom that had a home birth, breastfed for 4 years, co-slept, let my child feed herself, did "infant potty training" with her, delayed vaccinations and sent her to Montessori school. No homeschooling though.. not for me. Why did I do these things? I did them because they FELT RIGHT to me.. because something *inside* of me told me they were the right things to do, regardless of the pressures and opinions of others.. and BOY, did others have opinions on these topics! Even political discussions don't get as heated as moms debating over common parenting practices! OMG. I felt SO compelled to make some of these choices that there was no way I could have made a different decision, no matter what anyone else said.

What came next? My career. I realized that I needed a new one. Then my husband. It quickly became clear that I needed a new one of those too. It was incredible how the speaking up of this "gut instinct" created a domino effect and my life completely transformed into something else that I would have NEVER seen coming. I wish this "voice" would have spoken up sooner!!! Then maybe I wouldn't have had to undo decisions (big decisions!) that I had made without the guide of my instincts.

So, what is this "voice" I speak of? It's actually not really a "voice" for me. It's a feeling. One that I am going to try very hard to describe. It's a knowing that I feel absolutely *positive* about something without having any reason *why*. I believe there is a reason that many call it a "gut" instinct. For me, the bodily sensation that sometimes accompanies it tends to be centralized to the upper stomach area, that soft area below where your sternum, or breastbone, stop. This is anatomically where your stomach is, but most people don't know that. What I experience is a pressure, a solidness, a sense of confidence and assuredness. It is not an uncomfortable or uneasy feeling in any way.

Discomfort is what I feel when I *don't* know, when I *don't* feel confident and assured. I get *uneasy* when I am about to make the **wrong** decision. So maybe sometimes, I only know the wrong way to go and I have to feel around for the right one. The one that *doesn't* feel uneasy. I've never actually had the chance to discuss what others who experience this "voice" have to say about it, what their experiences are like. I really need to do that! I am quite sure everyone's experiences are a little different. Until I wrote this book, I never actually tried to put it in words. I just took the easy way out, like my mom, and said, "I just know." And there is so much truth in that. I KNOW and I don't need to know why. You can have confidence in that. You are a grown, adult woman and you don't need to justify your decisions to anyone.

I'm going to go out on a limb and assume that some of you reading this book know what I am talking about and some don't. For those of you who do, I urge you to cultivate and to listen to what that inner voice has to say. Follow its lead, and don't be afraid. I have been following it for about the last 15 years and it has been an amazing journey, which has brought me to where I am now.

For those of you who are unsure as to what this "inner voice" is: this is where meditation and quieting down your life really becomes important. It is extremely hard to hear your internal voice when it is constantly being drowned out by the incessant noise around you. In case you haven't noticed, we live in a world where there is *constant* noise. It never stops. Even the friggin' gas pumps have TVs on them now.. to talk at you while you are pumping gas. ARGH. Other people are *always* telling you what you should think and do, so it's no wonder if you are struggling to think for yourself. You have to actually MAKE AN EFFORT to step away from it or else it is always there. And I am not even talking about just *sound* noise. Now many of us are *reading* the noise. On the internet and on social media. You HAVE to get away from it, away from everyone else's thoughts and opinions in order to hear your own.

I love my quiet mornings. My husband leaves for work, I get my daughter off to school, I have my morning jasmine green tea and I sit down to write in my journal. I just write down whatever I want: plans for the day, thoughts about this or that, how I feel physically, mentally, emotionally.. it is my time to connect with ME. When my husband is home, he needs noise from the second he wakes up in the morning. He grabs his phone and starts watching videos, flips on the TV or has to talk... silence is not his thing. And as a consequence, this is someone who is not in touch with his "inner voice." He struggles to take action and make decisions because he never "feels" what the right thing to do is. He's not in tune with his decision-making center because he is always drowning it out and letting other people decide how he feels. At least that is my opinion.

My advice: Find your voice. Your "gut." Your "intuition." God. "The Universe." It doesn't matter what you call it, but what it has to say is *profound*. So connect with it, listen to it, follow it. I am not going to lie. It can be scary and it may result in the deconstruction of parts of your life, as it did mine.. but sometimes you have to tear down old rickety structures, so you can build more solid ones that will withstand the test of time. And perhaps this is exactly what you need to do! Maybe this is the cause of that nagging anxiety or depression. Just maybe your "gut" is trying to tell you something!

You Don't Have to be the BEST to be Awesome

"Don't take failure personally.
Get your ego out of it, and your curiosity into it."
–Jen Sincero

I thought about this topic one morning during one of my swim practices. I originally hesitated joining my swim club because I thought I wasn't a "good enough" swimmer to join the "club." As I was swimming along, I was thinking about how I am FAR from the fastest swimmer in the club - definitely on the slower side - I wear my fins (flippers) all throughout practice, so I don't get left behind (which would mean missing intervals and I would end up doing my own thing in a sea of other people doing something else.) At swim practice, I can sometimes get to feeling like I'm not that great of a swimmer simply because I'm not "the best" in my group. Then I have to laugh when I compare myself (which you should NEVER do!! :-)) to the "non-swim club" population. I am actually an AWESOME swimmer. So, if you are going to do the dirty deed and compare yourself to others.. take note of whom you are using for comparison.. or better yet... don't do it at all! I know I am not the only one who felt this way when embarking on something new. MANY people are too intimidated to join organizations that would welcome them with open arms out of fear of feeling awkward by not being the best at everything right off the bat. Why we are so afraid of being "new" is beyond me considering that EVERYONE is new at some point. No one is born an expert in anything. But I have fallen victim to it many times too. So I can empathize. Maybe it is just a matter of protecting our fragile "egos," which are in fact, *fragile*. We worry too much about being judged or ridiculed, and are maybe scarred by events in our childhoods. But remember: actual *adults* really don't do that.. ridicule each other.. and if you find yourself in a place where they do, then I recommend finding a new place where you can surround yourself with people who have actually completed maturity.

If you are a competitive type, you may find it hard to hang with people who are better than you at something. Maybe you prefer the company of people who are not at your level because this makes you feel more powerful and therefore, more *comfortable*. The thing is, you are not growing if you are not challenging yourself and you are not *really* challenging yourself if you aren't spending time with people who are better than you at something. Ok, so maybe this makes you feel inferior and maybe that feeling makes you uncomfortable. That's OK. Because staying in our comfort zone is not what brings you that awesome life you want to have. If you have an inkling of a feeling inside of you that you want to learn something new or improve on a skill you already have, you'll need to step out of your comfort zone to do it. If you want to be something other than what you are, then you have to do something other than what you usually do!

Look at your life and pay close attention to those people whom you envy, those people in your life who almost make you mad and bitter because they are doing the things that, deep down, you really want to be doing too. The family that is always going on vacations or that colleague that got the promotion that you really wanted. Instead of judging and being bitter, I recommend that you become **curious** instead. Become friendly with these people and figure out how **you** can do what they are doing, how you can change or improve so that you can have the things you want too. They are not "better" people than you. They are just doing things *differently* than you.

And have some humility, for goodness' sake! It's OK to be "new." It's OK to ask questions, to be curious, to fumble, to make mistakes, to be the slowest runner in the group or to have no idea what your colleague was just talking about. We're all clueless sometimes and none of us are the best at everything we do, but that shouldn't deter us altogether from trying something new. Before you run, you must first learn to walk, right?? It is those new experiences that open new doors for us and improve the quality of our lives. You are awesome for even trying something new, regardless of the outcome! So, do me a favor and let go of the notion that you have to be an expert at something before you even try it.. that doesn't make any sense now, does it?? Just shut out all those naysaying thoughts, those fears that probably won't even come to fruition.. and just do it. Sign up for that class or that club that you've been eyeing and making excuses not to. I doubt you'll regret it!

Finding Joy

The time to enjoy your life is NOW. So many people are waiting until later.. putting off the most fun and enjoyable things in life until some predetermined time in the future. When you have more money? Summer? The kids' graduate? 5 years? Retirement? What if you don't make it that long? Or something else happens to completely derail you? No one is guaranteed another day. If you are just trudging through your days, day after day, week after week without doing anything that truly makes you feel happy and excited, *joyful*, then this is a real problem. Don't be surprised if you are struggling with anxiety, depression, irritability, poor sleep, lack of energy and chronic pain. Living beings need joy in their daily lives. Look around you at the animals that live among us. Do you not see the playfulness in your dogs, your cats, the squirrels and birds chasing each other around outside? All you see in our animal counterparts is joy, love, the need to eat, rest and keep warm. That is what their whole lives are about! And they remain healthy, without the aid of modern medicine (the less domesticated ones, anyways).

I know one thing that has always driven a spear of doubt into my pursuit of joy, or having fun.. money. I'm not entirely sure where it came from, but I have an extremely deep seated fear of running out of money. I know I am not alone. SO many Americans share this same fear. We think we need to hoard our money. Save it. Trade a bigger bank account for your joy. Stay home and on your devices instead of going out and spending money on things that bring you and your family joy. Really?? This is the American way! But this is the thing. Money itself doesn't really bring most people joy. Money buys *experiences* that bring people joy. And here's the other thing. You can ALWAYS make more money. But you can't make more *time.* You can't stop your kids from growing up at the speed of light, or stop your body from aging. Time goes by and you can NEVER GET IT BACK.

I just went through that moment of anxiety myself. Again. I desperately want to spend the afternoon downhill skiing with my husband and daughter... but money is a bit tight this month and weekend skiing is expensive! As my daughter gets older, it's getting harder and harder to find things to do together. She wants to do things with her friends more often than not and she's not much into the "cheaper" outdoor activities, like hiking and XC skiing. My husband has also been having some trouble finding joy in his own life, I've noticed. I felt tormented for a couple of days over spending the money on an afternoon of skiing. It was uncomfortable for me to click that "Complete Purchase" button. But I did it anyway. My thoughts are this: I will NEVER regret spending that time with my two favorite people, laughing and goofing off and just generally having *fun.* I WILL regret watching more time pass by without doing that. I *will* regret, when my daughter goes off into the world, that I didn't grasp every possible opportunity to spend time with her that I could. No price can be put on that. In fact, my daughter gave me a really great compliment a couple of weeks ago. She said, "You know, Mom: I'm, like, the only person my age I know that actually *gets along* with my parents." At almost 14, I am definitely really glad she feels that way. I certainly like to think that's partly because I make an effort and spend money on experiences that allow us to be joyful and have fun together. The ironic thing is that I had to go through the same thing again, right after I bought the ski tickets, when I realized that a payment was due towards the vacation that we are taking in a couple of weeks. It was easier then.. I had already rationalized my way through the first action of giving away my money. If this money thing is an issue for you too, I recommend doing some research and working on shifting your mindset from that of "scarcity" to "abundance." There are a lot of great authors and speakers that talk about the importance of shifting your thinking from "there's never enough" (scarcity) to "there's always enough and there always will be" (abundance). I seem to gravitate towards these types of books, so I find them all the time! If you are curious, go into your search engine and type "abundance mindset." It may completely change you if you're open to it.

Do you need money to find joy? Absolutely not! I just love to travel, to be outside and to move my body so I spend money on travel expenses, gear and equipment. And books. My graduate degree? Mmmmm... that was a bit expensive.. but do I regret it? Heck, no!! So maybe I am paying for it until I die... oh well! What kind of price can you put on loving to go work?? My work actually brings me joy. Most activities require some kind of monetary contribution, but people are SUPER creative creatures, and there is more than one way to get what you want. Money is not always the vector!! We just seem to think it is, but we are mistaken.

If you find yourself trudging joylessly through your days, then I recommend thinking about ways to get some of it back. You are allowed to take time for yourself! What kinds of things excite you and make you feel alive? If you are a mom, you don't need to feel guilty about taking time for yourself. Do you want to teach your children that it's not OK for them to take time for themselves, that they should skip their own joy for the sake of someone else? If you take time out for yourself, they will *learn* from you to do it for themselves. If you don't, they will not do it either. We all want our kids to be happy. Why don't we allow the same for ourselves?

If you are having trouble finding things that bring you joy, maybe you can start by eliminating things that you know DON'T bring you joy... or take your joy away... things I call "joy thieves" or "energy vampires." If you do know what you can do to increase joy, do more of that AND do more eliminating! Maybe you are in a pretty good mood and then you watch the nightly news and suddenly you are filled with anxiety and dread. You can't sleep that night because your mind and heart won't stop racing. Is it possible that certain people or activities are actually *stealing* your joy away? I limit my interaction with news sources and social media.. and even now I started to shift my TV watching away from dark and depressing themes. I find that I am much happier that way. I take the "ostrich" route and bury my head in the sand when it comes to matters that I really can't change. Like politics? Why bother being anxious, angry and frustrated when I can't do a damn thing to change the situation that's causing it? I'd rather be happy and joyful if I can't change it. People are great at stealing your joy too. I try to limit my interaction with them as well. In some cases, you cannot fully escape, but you can limit the time spent with them. If you are happier and more joyful, you WILL attract more people and ideas that bring you joy. You will. I promise!!

Tools For Improving Mental Health

Anything that you do that increases joy in your life is going to help to improve your mental health. That's a given. In addition to pursuing your own activities (or maybe you are struggling to find some), I thought I would mention some tools that either I use or that I know others use and find helpful. Depending on where you are in your quest for self improvement, I recommend FIRST: improving your diet, SECOND: engaging in regular exercise and THEN adding in some of these other recommendations as needed. Improving diet and exercise quality will go a long way in improving mental health and are the two MOST important things to do for yourself. If you are struggling with time, I realize that those two alone can be a challenge for most busy women. You can actually combine some of these other ideas with exercise, such as exercising outdoors, while reading or listening to podcasts, or listening to podcasts while you are cooking healthy meals. I'm all about multitasking! Here's a few more things I think are important:

Quiet Time

There is a lot to be said for just taking even a few minutes out of your day to just be in the quiet, to let your mind catch up and stop reeling from all the noise and activity that happens around us on a daily basis. Part of what keeps me sane and focused on a daily basis is my morning "routine," which includes quiet time until I am ready to face the world. I wake up, I let my dogs out, I make tea and I drink my tea while I write in my journal. My quiet time and my journal writing give me a chance to set my mind right for the day. It gives me a chance to unload any issues that may be unsettling and swirling around in my head, and to set my focus on the day ahead: what do I want to accomplish today or in the near future? I often make lists in it. I keep track of my mood, my menses and check in on the general state of my body and mind. If I am feeling negatively for some reason, I acknowledge it and this helps me shift into a more positive state. It's one of my favorite routines of the day, so much so, that when my husband is home on weekends - the one who needs noise immediately upon waking - it makes me a little crazy. The interruption of my quiet time before I'm ready definitely makes me irritable. I have set up a small room in my house, my own little place to retreat to when everyone else needs noise and I need quiet.

I'm an introvert by nature, so I need more quiet time than most people. I like to think and reflect, and noise often prevents me from doing that. As I mentioned earlier, I cannot sense what I need or grow as a person without spending a lot of time with myself. I get tired, too, if I have a particularly busy day even if it isn't overly strenuous. Being around people is strenuous on my mind. My husband and I are polar opposites in this regard. He gets energized by being around people. I get exhausted. You'll probably see me try to slink away when my husband starts a conversation with a total stranger. But for me, this feeling of fatigue is exactly the same from mental stress as it is from physical stress. I just need to check out for a bit. If possible, I will take 20-30 minutes and just lay down in the quiet in the afternoon just to rest, reset and calm my nervous system. Or I may take a walk if I don't have the quiet space to rest. It has taken me many years to realize that I need this in order to remain a pleasant person. I remember when my daughter was tiny.. I would take her to these places to play that were so busy and noisy, and she and I both would be so exhausted afterwards. I would say "oh, she's just overstimulated" and had no idea why I was so tired.. I was clearly "overstimulated" too! Overstimulation means irritability for me if I don't deal with it. I've come to learn that. I've used alcohol in the past to cope with said irritability. Now I just try to listen to my body's cues and use a more preventative approach. I check out for a bit when I feel that "people" fatigue coming on.

If you have a particularly busy life or schedule, I recommend trying to carve out maybe 20 minutes a day for either quiet or meditation. Meditation (addressed below) is the same sort of "rest" time, only it's more focused, more actively redirecting your mind away from the busy thoughts. Some people have more trouble turning their thoughts off and settling their nervous system without some help. Or it just might be more convenient to sit and listen to a meditation on some earbuds on your phone than to find a place to rest, depending on your daily activities. You can even just go for a quiet walk, if you can get away. Either way, you will give your mind a much needed mental "break".. and your body too! Because if your mind is stressed, trust me.. your body is feeling it too!

Your entire being NEEDS mental rest for the sake of your health. Living in a state where you are constantly amped up is just not a good thing. You will burn yourself out, and burnt out can be a very hard thing to recover from, depending on the severity. When we thing of "burn out," we think mentally, right? "Burn out" doesn't only affect the mental body.. since we have already discussed the fact that the body and mind are not separate... your physical body will be damaged also. And it's entirely possible that this damage becomes irreparable, the longer you go without taking proper care of yourself. The best treatment is prevention. So start now.

Mental Health Counseling

I truly think that everyone can benefit from the help of a good mental health counselor. I consider this *maintenance*, and no one should even need to feel ashamed to seek mental health counseling. We ALL have issues that can addressed, whether it's from childhood, problematic relationships, work-related or other personal concerns. We can ALWAYS do better at handling ourselves in certain situations and in being more empathetic towards others, and ourselves! Mental health counselors are skilled at teaching coping mechanisms for various mental health issues and also at helping to put patients' issues into a better perspective and encouraging a change in thought patterns. Sometimes a change in perspective and/or a few good techniques (with practice!) is all one needs to combat issues like stress, chronic irritability, anxiety and depression. Even just having an uninterrupted, non-biased ear to listen to your issues and concerns can go a very long way. In more serious cases, medication can be helpful, but I am a believer that one should seek all possible alternatives before settling on the medication route and still actively engage in learning better coping techniques and thought patterns. Medication often does not 100% take care of the issues, so this is necessary anyway.

A few years ago, I sought the help of a mental health counselor to help me cope with anxiety and the overconsumption of alcohol. I had started to feel like alcohol was taking over my life, almost like I couldn't imagine my life without it. It was major coping mechanism for my anxiety and I didn't know how I'd be able to function without it in my life. I may have already mentioned this, but I began having panic attacks when I was 22, when one attack came absolutely out of nowhere. I didn't even know what it was at the time and it scared me. A LOT. Since that time, I have battled bouts of panic and anxiety, although I have mostly gotten the panic attacks under control. I still sometimes feel that "rush," my heart speeds up and the adrenaline starts pumping through my body, but I no longer freak out about it. It's like a wave that comes on, and I know in a few minutes it will have passed. And it does. It always does. They started to pass when I started working with a mental health counselor, one who offered me techniques, things that I could do in the moment to help keep the attacks under control. Over the course of the next couple of years, I worked to also get my anxiety under better control and, at the time of writing this very section, I am now 61 days alcohol-free. (And have since noticed that the alcohol was a contributing factor to my anxiety. It was actually making it worse, not better!). It takes some work and a willingness to be introspective, to have some humility so that changes can be made. We can all be better, so why not try?

With that said, it is important to find someone who you feel is right for you. Who helps you to feel better and not worse. I was fortunate to get one that I really like right off the bat.. and although I am doing really well, I still like to see her regularly. I find being able to "unload" extremely therapeutic all by itself, as it is not something I do regularly. I am a private person by nature, and I do not feel right burdening others with my "problems." If you aren't fortunate to find someone you like right away, keep looking. I swear it is worth it! Especially if you feel like your mental health issues are getting in the way of doing the things you love. I love to travel, but the actual process of "traveling" gives me terrible anxiety. I LOVE planning, but the actual process of getting from point A to point B.. especially if it involves an airplane.. Oi. I'm crazy uptight until I get to the destination. But to me, it's a necessary evil, as I am not willing to give up my dreams to travel anywhere and everywhere I can. I am also unwilling to medicate. SO that means figuring out ways to cope. Which brings me to the next section, as it is another one of my favorite mental health boosters: meditation (with a "T", not a "C").

Meditation

I sometimes have to engage in some form of "meditation" when I feel especially stressed and anxious. Meditation is a form of mental "rest" that I mentioned earlier. It's like hitting the RESET button in your brain. When we get stressed/anxious, it's like our mind starts going berserk: thoughts starts racing (usually unpleasant ones), which then elicit uncomfortable sensations in the body, like a tight chest and throat, shortness of breath, racing heart, extremity numbness, a feeling of being trapped in our bodies when maybe we want to leave! But guess what? We can't...

Meditation isn't just sitting cross-legged on the floor with your eyes closed and zoning out, thinking no thoughts, like it is depicted in movies. You can sit, lie down or even take a walk in the woods (my favorite!). Meditation is actually just practicing exercises to retrain your mind in a setting where you can remain undistracted by certain elements of the outside world, elements that distract you from being able to focus on your own thoughts. It's time cut out specifically to "hear yourself think." Ever heard that expression? It's such a MOM thing to say, isn't it?? "I CAN'T HEAR MYSELF THINK!!" But as a 44-year old mom, I totally get it. I need to take time regularly to "hear myself think" or else I go bananas! (I actually find it quite ridiculous that we have to MAKE TIME to do this – this is how constantly distracting our lives actually are).

There are MANY different forms of meditation. There is something called *guided* meditation, where someone else speaks and *guides* you to think thoughts that relax you and make you feel more positive. There are apps for your phone that can do this, as well as trained people in your community that you can seek out if you are interested in pursuing something like this. If you are the type who, when you sit or lie down quietly, you can't stop your mind from racing, this would benefit you greatly. There is also *visual* meditation, which is a form of meditation in which you are looking and focusing on an object. You can do this with sound too. Listening to music can actually be a form of meditation, also, as it allows you to calm your mind. Obviously, this only applies if the music is soothing. Exercise can be meditative too, depending on what you are doing and where. I find walking in the woods to be extremely soothing. Sometimes I get stressed in my house - too much to do or too many people around - so seek quiet away from home. The woods provides that place for me. It could be a park, a beach or even just your back yard.

The ability to calm your mind is a skill that requires cultivation. Practice. If you are not the type to ever try, you may find it quite difficult at first. It's important to practice it regularly to really reap the benefits. But you have to know... it really isn't that complicated! If you lead an especially busy or hectic life, you really just need to take a few minutes, ideally a half hour, to STOP running around and filling your ears with our cultural noise, so you can connect with your own thoughts, your own inner voice and your own body. It's extremely important for the wellness of our bodies and our minds.

Reading/Listening to Podcasts

I personally love to read and listen to positive and motivating books and podcasts. There are periods in my life during which I get stuck in "mental ruts." I feel like I am not moving forward - I hate staying still, not just physically, but mentally and spiritually too. I will feel frustrated and apathetic, and even the things I normally do to bring me joy don't work. Then I get even more frustrated. Oftentimes, a motivating book or podcast will help kick me out of it. To be honest, books and podcasts are solely responsible for changing my view on and my relationship with money. Maybe that sounds unrelated, but at one point, I realized that my view on money was a major obstacle for me to to pursue the things I really wanted. That was pretty seriously affecting my mental health. There are some really great motivational people out there. My favorites are Tony Robbins, James Wedmore (business), Jen Sincero, Brene Brown, Robert Kiyosaki (money).. the teachings of these people have honestly helped transform my thoughts, my relationships, my decisions and ultimately, my life. If you don't do much of this, and you don't know where to start, I highly recommend reading (or listening to!) *The Four Agreements*, by Don Miguel Ruiz. This was the very first book I read while on my path to self improvement, and it completely transformed by relationships and my thoughts around myself and others. It is small, but mighty!

The great thing about audiobooks and podcasts is that you can listen to them while you are out and about. I don't often take the time to sit and read books. If I am sitting, I am usually writing.. but I do spend enough time in a car.. so I can easily pull up podcasts or audiobooks on my phone and listen to them while I am driving.

Just pick one and get started. It may just give you the jumpstart that you need.

The Great Outdoors

Oh, how I love to be outside! I've come to realize that the places where I am happiest is in "wide open spaces." I get stressed and anxious when I am cramped, stuck inside small spaces.. even a house. I need out. I need nature to stay sane.

One of my favorite things to do is to hike the Adirondack mountains, and I have spent much time reflecting on why. I mean, I spend half a day walking up a mountain and the other half walking down. It's hard work! I can see why my passion for this hobby puzzles people. I've come to realize that spending an entire day within the confines of only nature is like a mental reset for me. It is an experience unlike any other ones in my life. And there's a very specific reason that I choose the difficult experiences, not the easy walks in the woods. 1- It gives me a sense of accomplishment, and 2- It takes a long time, so I spend an entire day (or sometimes longer) detached from the usual demands of life and in nature, mostly just with myself and my husband, and in my own mind. Don't get me wrong, it isn't easy, physically or mentally. As I mentioned earlier, getting out of my comfort zone is something I try to do regularly. I have completed enough strenuous activities to know that my mind constantly cycles between anxiety and enjoyment. I never *not* feel some modicum of fear and anxiety when embarking on a new adventure, whether it be hiking or otherwise. My anxiety tries to be debilitating and stop me from doing the things I really want to be doing, but I work really hard not to let it. When I don't let it win and I accomplish what I set out to do, I feel VERY empowered and then I become more confident in my ability to overcome it in the future. Hiking the mountains is very therapeutic for me because it gives me the time I need in the "wide open spaces" (you don't get more wide or open than standing on top of a mountain top!), away from noisy distractions and listening to everyone else's opinion, and in the end, leaves me feeling strong, confident and empowered. I can't say that many other experiences in my life can equal that.

Building Your Own Wellness Gauge

S o now that we are getting close to wrapping this up, I want to circle back to the very first question I asked you when this book began: "Is my body properly nourished?" The thing is, in order to answer this question, you need to also ask yourself this secondary question, "How do I *know* if my body is properly nourished?" What is your "gauge" for knowing whether or not you are well, or healthy? I challenge you to look inside yourself for this answer. If you are basing your judgement on tests and exams performed by people who hardly ever see you, and all the while you are struggling with chronic, ongoing discomfort in your life, like pain, mood instability, debilitating anxiety, sleep issues, digestive issues, etc, then I *definitely* urge you to rethink your position. I can't tell you the number of patients I've seen whose doctors have deemed them perfectly "healthy," but who suffer from chronic migraines, digestive issues, menstrual pain & other chronic pain, anxiety/depression/panic attacks, sleeplessness, fatigue, all of unknown origin. The medical doctors can't find the cause, and so they tell them there isn't one, that they are "fine," when they are, in fact, NOT FINE. I have had to reassure many patients by letting them know that there IS a cause and just because the doctors can't find it doesn't mean there ISN'T something wrong. People know instinctively when their bodies are not functioning the way they usually do, and I have seen the amount of anguish and frustration that comes from patients who are suffering and after test after test, the medical doctors tell them that "nothing is wrong." Something is wrong for this patient to even be in your office!!! I have even talked to patients whose doctors have referred them to psychologists because the doctors told them it must be "all in their head." Heartbreaking!!!

Obviously, I operate from a totally different paradigm. Any one that walks into my office seeking my care is off balance in some way, and they know it, even when they are often told everything is "fine." Otherwise, they wouldn't be there! Most have pain that won't go away or other chronic issues that are ill-managed by other treatment options. Acupuncture and Chinese medicine are often at the bottom of list of treatment options for most people, and they only seek care when nothing else has worked. I would like to see this shift and for these therapies to fall higher up on the list of treatment options. The reason is this: *most* chronic issues that cannot be treated by mainstream medicine are issues of deficiency. Meaning: something important is missing inside the patient's body and this is why the body is malfunctioning. Unless this underlying deficiency is addressed, no amount of medications or surgeries are going to ever *solve* the problem. Mask it, yes. Alleviate it, maybe. But NOT fix it. In some cases, it may be a genetic condition in which the patient is actually just not born with all the required mechanics. Type I diabetes, for example. Some people's bodies are born without the ability to make insulin, and so they need a management plan for the rest of their lives. But in MOST cases, chronic issues in the body (especially those that come on later in life) develop in response to an internal deficiency of some sort.

Modern medicine is absolutely amazing in so many ways, but I have to be honest.. there's really still A LOT that is unknown. Our bodies are extremely complex and our ability to test and image them while they are living and moving is still quite limited. On the other hand, Chinese medicine is ancient. It has been around for thousands of years, but it is a bit more archaic. The bulk of Chinese medical theory was created before technology, before the ability to analyze blood and take detailed images of the body. It is based on thousands of years of watching the body operate from a non-invasive standpoint and from listening to patients during this time. Chinese medicine bases much of its diagnostic platform on what the patients say (it puts THAT kind of trust in the patients); Western medicine practitioners use more objective test results as the basis of their diagnoses. Western medicine and Chinese medicine actually make a really great pair; you could say that they are the yin & yang of medicine.

They are synergistic and not oppositional.

With that said, when it comes to your own wellness, the most important thing you can do is to trust your own body, as you alone know your body better than anyone else. Chronic ailments and debilitating mood changes are NOT a sign of wellness. I have seen patients who have spent years of their life struggling with unmanaged conditions. You don't need to do this! If you *know* in your gut that something is off, trust it. Remember we talked about that? Seek other types of care, and don't stop until you feel better. There are so many other places to look. There are many different types of bodyworkers: acupuncturists, chiropractors, massage therapists, physical therapists, yoga therapists... and there are just as many different types of mental health practitioners and support groups that can offer care. But remember: You must ALSO be willing to make lifestyle changes, as in many cases, no one can actually make you feel better but YOU. YOU have to deal with faults in your diet. YOU have to figure out a way to move your body more if you're not. YOU have to acknowledge and accept emotional and mental blockages that may be hindering progress or causing you to turn to behaviors that are sabotaging your efforts. I know this probably seems very overwhelming, but there are SO MANY people and organizations out there that can help you do this. And all you have to do is literally log onto your computer or pick up your phone to find them. Start with one that seems appealing, that you've thought about or maybe even someone you know. Once you take that step, you will most assuredly be on your way.

Here are some examples of my own wellness gauges:

My bowel movements. Bowel movements are a great assessment of digestive health. As a Chinese medicine practitioner, I will sometimes ask a lot of questions about a patient's bowel movements, which sometimes catches them off guard. After all, this isn't a topic that we discuss regularly.. or even realize that it's important! But it is. Your bowel movements are basically a reflection on how well your body is digesting the food you are putting in, and how your body is responding to it. They should be happening almost daily, and they should be firm and formed, easy to pass and not painful. This is the ideal. If you are regularly constipated, have loose and unformed stools or experience pain, I would consider making some dietary changes. Food sensitivities are the #1 culprit of intestinal irregularities. When my diet is on, which is basically full on "paleo" (grain-free) these days, my bowel movements are PERFECT.. And that actually makes me happy because then I know I am doing the right thing for my body. I can actually tell that my body doesn't like grains that much because consuming them causes my bowels to change. I become constipated, irregular and inconsistent.

My menses. The menstrual cycle is another solid gauge of overall wellness. Assessing your menstrual cycle can tell you a lot about your liver function and the quality and quantity of your blood. Think about how important your blood is. Our blood is what carries nourishment to every square inch of our bodies. It carries much needed oxygen to our organs, our brains, our skeletal tissues. It is also what brings elements required to repair damage. When we cut our finger, it is the elements contained in our blood that prevents the cut from getting infected and begins the process of healing the wound. Yet, in Western medicine, not much emphasis is placed on assessing the *health* of our blood. Sure, doctors take a look at certain markers, but it is still a highly fragmented method, and in my opinion, is not an adequate was to holistically assess blood health. *Blood deficiency* is an extremely common pattern seen in women from a Chinese medicine perspective. It means that their blood is not adequately nourishing their body. Either they simply don't have enough blood to go around, or the blood that they do have is not as healthy as it could be.

These are issues you can easily spot when assessing your own menstrual cycle. The ideal menstrual cycle should be smooth and regular, not painful and the amount of blood should be neither too little or too much. Experiencing pain, mood changes, digestive or sleep issues around ovulation and/or menses or completely irregular cycles means your liver is struggling to process the hormonal changes and you could benefit from being kinder to your liver (less stress, less medication/drugs and alcohol, and dietary improvements can help your liver tremendously. If you are regularly bleeding heavily, this is not good, and if you are barely bleeding at all, this is a problem too. A healthy menstrual cycle indicates good circulation. If yours is disordered, you may want to think about investigating ways to improve it.

My level of inner peace. Rising anxiety levels are an indicator that I need to make some changes, be it physical, mental or emotional. This is a definitely a bit trickier, as anxiety manifests for MANY different reasons. It can physical, mental, emotional, menstrual-cycle related, situational. I have spent a great deal of time working to get in touch with my anxiety triggers. Sometimes I can eliminate or reduce them, and sometimes I just have to deal with the anxiety because I simply can't avoid them. In any case, if I find myself experiencing prolonged anxiety for reasons I can't specify, then I start to evaluate and make changes.

One gauge I use on my patients is to assess their use of over-the-counter (OTC) and prescription medications. I've had countless patients report that they have no issues in certain areas, but then their medication list tells me a different story. If you are regularly taking OTC meds (like ibuprofen, acetaminophen, TUMs, etc) or a daily medication for management of some conditions, then you STILL have issues that need work, in my opinion. Taking daily medication may mean that your issue is "managed," but it is certainly not solved if you need to continue to take it. Taking daily medication is not ideal for your body.

It's a process. It's a long and windy road, and there will be bumps and blockages. You will have to reroute and double back sometimes, but that's totally normal. Just get back on the road. One thing at a time. One day at a time. DON'T GIVE UP ON YOURSELF. You have a whole lifetime to work on it, but it's so worth it. You're worth it. Our young women, who can be taught early on to care for themselves so they don't have to suffer, are worth it.

Epilogue

Many people have asked me, "How do you do so much?" I attribute my health, my productivity, and my excitement about life to all of things that I have described in this book. I am not gifted in any way, or superhuman. I am just a person who is curious and loves to learn, especially when it comes to the human body, health and healing. Sometime during my mid-20s, I became obsessed with health and wellness. I have not stopped researching and learning about it over the past 20 years, so this book is a condensed cultivation of the things I know, the things that have contributed to my ongoing ability and desire to keep learning, growing and seeking out new adventures.

Since writing the bulk of this book, I decided to *mostly* end my relationship with alcohol (special occasions only!), as I couldn't shake the nagging feeling that I was continually doing damage to my body. I finally got off that "roller coaster," and it was one of the best decisions I ever made. No more mental torment, anxiety, hangovers, feeling bad about myself. My relationship with it was a long and tumultuous, good times, bad times and times in between. But it was time to end it and I had known that for awhile. At 45, it's time to start thinking about longevity. I plan to make it to 100!

I hope that my readers find value in this book. I **truly** want to help women improve the quality of their lives but the reach in my own practice is so limited. So my goal is to get this book into the hands of as many women as possible. I hope that it has helped you in even the smallest way, because all it takes sometimes is one small nudge to get the momentum for change rolling. If it has helped you, please pass it along.

Thanks for reading!

References

Bawa AS, Anilakumar KR. Genetically modified foods: safety, risks and public concerns-a review. *J Food Sci Technol.* 2013;50(6):1035-1046. doi:10.1007/s13197-012-0899-1

Chapman BP, Fiscella K, Kawachi I, Duberstein P, Muennig P. Emotion suppression and mortality risk over a 12-year follow-up. *J Psychosom Res.* 2013;75(4):381-385. doi:10.1016/j.jpsychores.2013.07.014

Edmunds, Theresa. Food for thought: Growing gluten intolerance stems from hybridized wheat:
https://www.thenewsherald.com/downriver_life/life/
food-for-thought-growing-gluten-intolerance-stems-from-hybridized-wheat/
article_e71b00d6-4fd5-528e-a16f-2c061e5cf1ec.html#:~:text=
Wheat%20has%20been%20hybridized%20during,study%20found%2014%
20new%20ones. (2013)

Eisenhauer B, Natoli S, Liew G, Flood VM. Lutein and Zeaxanthin-Food Sources, Bioavailability and Dietary Variety in Age-Related Macular Degeneration Protection. *Nutrients.* 2017;9(2):120. Published 2017 Feb 9. doi:10.3390/nu9020120

Gang-Jee Ko, Connie M. Rhee, Kamyar Kalantar-Zadeh, Shivam Joshi. The Effects of High-Protein Diets on Kidney Health and Longevity. *JASN* Aug 2020, 31 (8) 1667-1679; **DOI:** 10.1681/ASN.2020010028

Graham BM, Denson TF, Barnett J, Calderwood C, Grisham JR. Sex Hormones Are Associated With Rumination and Interact With Emotion Regulation Strategy Choice to Predict Negative Affect in Women Following a Sad Mood Induction. *Front Psychol.* 2018;9:937. Published 2018 Jun 11. doi:10.3389/fpsyg.2018.00937

Hallberg O, Johansson O. Comparing lung cancer risks in sweden, USA, and Japan. *ISRN Oncol.* 2012;2012:687298. doi:10.5402/2012/687298

Haug A, Høstmark AT, Harstad OM. Bovine milk in human nutrition—a review. *Lipids Health Dis.* 2007;6:25. Published 2007 Sep 25. doi:10.1186/1476-511X-6-25

He K, Li X, Chen X, et al. Evaluation of antidiabetic potential of selected traditional Chinese medicines in STZ-induced diabetic mice. J Ethnopharmacol. 2011;137(3):1135–1142.

Johnson EJ. The role of carotenoids in human health. *Nutr Clin Care.* 2002;5(2):56-65. doi:10.1046/j.1523-5408.2002.00004.x

Kennedy D. O. (2016). B Vitamins and the Brain: Mechanisms, Dose and Efficacy—A Review. *Nutrients, 8*(2), 68. doi:10.3390/nu8020068

Khoo HE, Azlan A, Tang ST, Lim SM. Anthocyanidins and anthocyanins: colored pigments as food, pharmaceutical ingredients, and the potential health benefits. *Food Nutr Res.* 2017;61(1):1361779. Published 2017 Aug 13. doi:10.1080/16546628.2017.1361779

Kumle M, Weiderpass E, Braaten T, Persson I, Adami HO, Lund E. Use of oral contraceptives and breast cancer risk: The Norwegian-Swedish Women's Lifestyle and Health Cohort Study. Cancer Epidemiol Biomarkers Prev. 2002 Nov;11(11):1375-81. PMID: 12433714.

MNT Editorial Team. Modern medicine: Infectious diseases, timelines, and challenges. Medical News Today. https://www.medicalnewstoday.com/articles/323538#where-are-we-now. Published November 2, 2018. Accessed February 28, 2021.

Muscle Pain: It May Actually Be Your Fascia. Johns Hopkins Medicine. https://www.hopkinsmedicine.org/health/wellness-and-prevention/muscle-pain-it-may-actually-be-your-fascia. Accessed March 5, 2021.

Negrini D, Moriondo A. Lymphatic anatomy and biomechanics. *J Physiol.* 2011;589(Pt 12):2927-2934. doi:10.1113/jphysiol.2011.206672

Nuttall FQ. Body Mass Index: Obesity, BMI, and Health: A Critical Review. *Nutr Today.* 2015;50(3):117-128. doi:10.1097/NT.0000000000000092

Santín-Márquez R, Alarcón-Aguilar A, López-Diazguerrero NE, Chondrogianni N, Königsberg M. Sulforaphane - role in aging and neurodegeneration. *Geroscience.* 2019;41(5):655-670. doi:10.1007/s11357-019-00061-7

Smith, MD, Robert C, 2018 (https://www.psychologytoday.com/us/blog/patient-zero/201808/rene-descartes-villain-or-savior-mental-health-care)

Story EN, Kopec RE, Schwartz SJ, Harris GK. An update on the health effects of tomato lycopene. *Annu Rev Food Sci Technol.* 2010;1:189–210. doi:10.1146/annurev.food.102308.124120

Other resources:

Ace Fitness: https://www.acefitness.org/education-and-resources/lifestyle/blog/5078/how-to-eat-and-train-for-an-endomorph-body-type/

"The Fuzz Speech" by Gil Hedley: https://www.youtube.com/watch?v=_FtSPtkSug

High Sugar Levels Increase Cancer and Mortality Risk: Jan 2005, https://www.jh-sph.edu/news/news-releases/2005/samet-blood-sugar.html#:~:text=Ele-vated%20blood%20sugar%20levels%20and,Yonsei%20University%20in%20Seoul%2C%20Korea

Cancer Cells Feed on Sugar-Free Diet: Study highlights role of glutamine in absence of glucose in growth of B cell tumors, Jan 2012: https://www.hop-kinsmedicine.org/news/media/releases/cancer_cells_feed_on_sugar_free_diet

The Nephron Information Center: http://nephron.org/nephsites/adp/pro-tein_ckd.htm

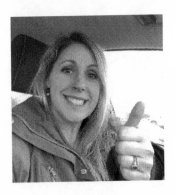

About the Author

Dr. Adrienne J. Goodman-LaMora, L.Ac., is the owner of *Longevity Complementary Care Center* in Macedon, NY, where she has successfully treated hundreds of patients using Traditional Chinese medicine. Adrienne holds a doctorate in Acupuncture & Chinese medicine and has been practicing this phenomenal medicine for over 10 years. Adrienne specializes in women's health and sports-related injuries. She is a triathlete and self-taught nutrition expert. In 2019, she completed her first full-distance triathlon. She currently resides in Palmyra, NY with her husband (Matt), daughter (Anna) and two dogs (Spike & Missy).

You can connect with me on:
- http://acupuncturingathlete.com
- https://www.facebook.com/adriennelamoraauthor

Also by Adrienne J. Goodman-LaMora, DACM, L.Ac.

Adrienne maintains a blog at:
   http://acupuncturingathlete.com/

Hope to see you there!

Made in the USA
Middletown, DE
26 April 2021